FOOD FOR THE SOUL

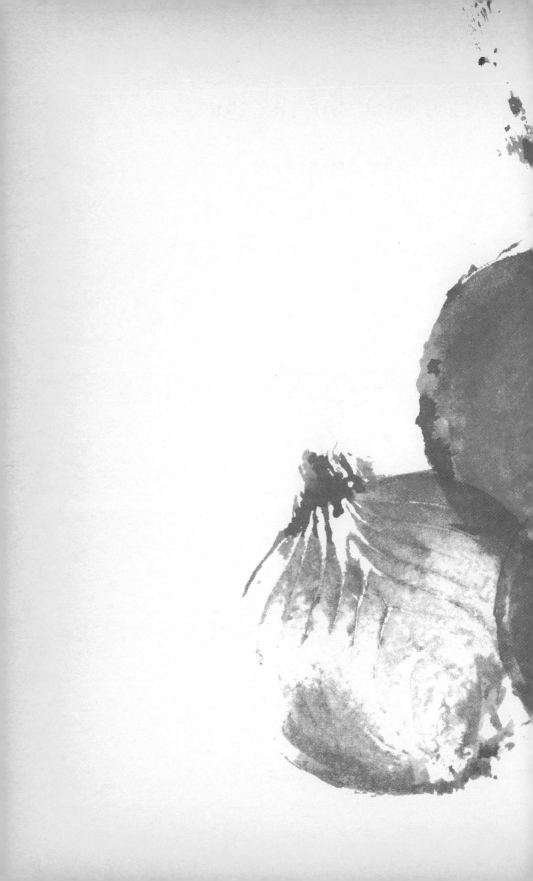

FOOD FOR THE SOUL

RECIPES FROM A KITCHEN TEMPLE

By

Manuela Dunn Mascetti and Arunima Borthwick

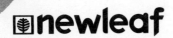

ADVICE TO THE READER

*Before following any medical or dietary advice
contained in this book, it is recommended that
you consult your doctor if you suffer from any
health problems or special conditions or are in
any doubt as to its suitability.*

First published 1997 by Newleaf, an
imprint of Macmillan Publishers Ltd, 25
Eccleston Place, London, SW1W 9NF
and Basingstoke.

Associated companies throughout the
world

ISBN 0 7522 0547 1

1 3 5 7 9 10 8 6 4 2
A CIP catalogue entry for this book is
available from the British Library

Typeset by SX Composing DTP,
Rayleigh, Essex
Printed and bound in Great Britain by
The Bath Press, Bath
Designed by DW Design
Original illustrations © Avesh

CONTENTS

III. HARMONY BETWEEN BODY AND SOUL

Dedication

For Osho

Acknowledgements

This book would never have been born, had it not been for the gentle but persistent encouragement of our publisher, Michael Alcock. He was the first to recognise the soul-quality of our candle-lit dinners and to offer his enthusiastic support throughout the conception and the writing. Thank you for fathering this creation into life.

The enchanted world of Osho is the true spirit that blesses this work. Sitting with Him in meditation, and spending time in His beautiful commune in Pune, India, is what has truly enabled the flower He gave us to shed its fragrance in our daily lives. Our deep gratitude is to Him and to all those sannyasins who continue undaunted in the work he set before us.

Thank you to the friendly spirits that have helped in the making of this book: Julie Foakes and Rowie Jackson for so lovingly typing the manuscript, and to Vicky Monk for her editorial supervision.

Thank you to Osho International Foundation for allowing us to enrich the text with Osho's original words and meditations.

And, finally, thank you to P and M for loving us more every day.

{Babette} had the ability to transform a dinner into a kind of love affair. A love affair that made no distinction between bodily appetite and spiritual appetite...

– Isak Dinesen, from Babette's Feast

INTRODUCTION

Practise random acts of kindness
And senseless acts of beauty.

—Anne Herbert

In the time of the Indian saint Mahavira, his Jain monks would sweep the path before them with brooms, and they would do this whenever they walked because they believed that every living thing, plant or animal, was a soul waiting to be reincarnated into human consciousness; to kill it by mistake, to kill it unconsciously, was to interfere with its karmic process. The Jain attitude to non-violence might seem extreme to Westerners, but it underscores an enchantment with the world: if the world has a soul, then the world is a soul-mate and a lover, and thus it is part of ourselves. As children we are read fairytales, the main characters of which are animals leading real lives parallel to our own; the enchantment of childhood is in believing that everything outside us is like us, alive and inhabited by soul. The awe and respect for the world that childhood and sainthood share become distorted when our thoughts and actions fail to respect not only that vital bond with our environment, but fail to care for our bodies also. Eating is ingesting parts of the world; if this was firmly lodged into our memories when we set out to prepare a meal, what kind of food would we choose? Perhaps we would not want to eat the result of killing. Instead, we might choose products that are naturally derived from the earth.

Throughout Asian countries, from India to Thailand, certain days are dedicated to sharing the bounty of earth with all its living forms; there are festivals for feeding pigeons, sea celebrations, when adults and children alike feed the fish; festivals in which the favourite foods of the gods are prepared and given in offering before their statues. Traditionally vegetarian, Asia honours the abundance of the planet in thousands of ways every day of the year.

Food for the Soul is an invitation to participate in the sacred dimension of cooking and eating the bounty that Nature offers us. Today, a vegetarian diet no longer means the adoption of austerity and a strict regime; blessed as we are with plenty, we can feast every day with an extraordinary array of produce which has been organically grown to respect the environment and to protect us from the harmful effects of pesticides and chemical fertilisers. *Food for the Soul* is also an open invitation for all of us to start caring for our planet in the same way we care for our body in whatever small and grand ways we can practically manage. We are now in the latter quarter of the twentieth century when half of humanity appears to be dying from starvation and the other half seems to be choking on its own excess, and we are, individually, largely unaware of this condition and its effects on the planet.

Many of the recipes and the principles behind the book originate from temple life. Having spent years living in ashrams and communes, where the main focus is meditation, we feel that food which has been cultivated and prepared with awareness and love, with no expectation for personal gain, is the best food to nourish the soul. Vegetarian meals have the additional benefit of combining aesthetics with health; cooking with natural ingredients is a way of contemplating beauty and of offering a work of beauty to others – this is the giving and receiving which adds depth to everyday life. We suggest that you create a temple out of your kitchen too; take the time you spend there, from making breakfast to a simple cup of tea, as your time of spiritual retreat. Be slow, gentle, and pay attention to *what* you do and *how* you do it. The more meditative in your approach to nourishment, the less stressed, the more healed you will be – this is a natural and simple equation that does not fail. Allow your intuition and imagination to help you play with food and the serving of meals. However tired or restless you feel when you are about to start your cooking tasks, if your kitchen is a temple you will feel renewed and re-enchanted by your time spent there.

We hope you will enjoy the recipes and the meditations *Food for the Soul* offers you; and above all we hope that you too will gain insight into the sacredness of small gestures in everyday tasks.

SECTION | I

MAKING

the body a

TEMPLE

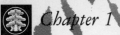

Chapter 1

Religion, Magic, Ritual & Food

The sacred dimension of preparing and eating food has been eclipsed in our homes, and yet these are actions that we perform daily, just like rituals in temples. We are fortunate indeed in being able to eat not only every day, but also in choosing from an incredible abundance of produce, yet we must remember that our lives are very different from that of a million others who are starving as we are eating. It is not the preciousness of food that makes it sacred, although this has been a major influence in the past. Sacredness is a certain way of caring for *what* we eat and *how* we eat; it reveals attention, healing, value and heart. We do not use the word sacred in a religious context; it is rather a quality or a dimension of experiencing everyday actions. Valuing the sacredness of food means eating soulfully, which in turn implies that particular attention is given to what we choose to take from the outside in order to nourish the inside. In this simple osmosis we can either feel a sense of relating to the whole, or we can carry on the process automatically. The difference between these two attitudes is simple: a balance of health and harmony in the body, mind and spirit.

All eating can be seen as communion, feeding the soul as well as the body. Our cultural habit of opting for fast food

reflects our current belief that all we need to ingest is, both literally and figuratively, *any* food, not food of real substance shared with others in celebration at the dinner table. Most of our culture and science, physical and social, operates as if there were no interior life, or at least assumes that the interior life has little or nothing to do with the outside world. When the interior is acknowledged it is almost invariably regarded as secondary, to be attended to only after the business at hand of office, family and home. The contemporary philosopher Thomas Moore says, 'Culturally we have a plastic esophagus, suited perhaps to fast food and fast living, but not conducive to soul, which thrives only when life is taken in a long, slow process of digestion and absorption.'

Retrieving the sacred in our lives demands that we bring back enchantment into everyday actions and processes. Enchantment in our surroundings, for instance, can be found if we begin to think in terms of having a house for our bodies, a home for our hearts and a temple for our souls. The building – the place where we live – remains the same, but under the spell of enchantment, it is perceived as nurturing three very different, albeit equally important, functions. The same enchantment can be brought back to cooking and eating – these can be seen as the two magical functions of nourishing and healing our bodies. The kitchen then becomes a temple where, magically, raw food is alchemically transformed into a glorious substance that sustains us in all dimensions. The author Isak Dinesen, in her famous tale *Babette's Feast*, tells us how Babette, an apparently simple French cook in the service of two old Danish spinsters, spends the money won in a lottery to buy the most expensive food for a celebration dinner in honour of the sisters' late father. As a parishioner he had transformed with his eloquent sermons and selfless dedication the lives of all the members of the congregation who, upon his sudden death, feel abysmally lost and unguided. As the guests sit down for dinner we get a sense of the bitterness of their lives; nothing is happy, the joyous taste has left their spirit. Babette, who is revealed to be quite a witch, not only serves an outstanding meal, but her cooking has the power to transform the quality of the guests' hearts. It is as though they were eating the essence of the parishioner and so progressively they absorb his enlightenment into their bodies during the meal. At the end of the evening everyone feels pervaded by spiritual goodness and they leave the house wondering whether they have been transmuted into angels. Their transformation is symbolic of the rite of the Eucharist, in which the communicant is purified as the divine essence – in the form of blessed food – is digested.

Babette's Feast is a richly woven tale which imaginatively describes the transformative powers of food, but many more examples can be found in popular folk traditions. The witch's brew, the magic cauldron, the enchanted potion, the healing drink, the shaman's herbs for vision questing – these are all expressions of the timeless knowledge that food is not only for the body, but that it essentially nourishes the soul too. Britain and most of Asia have little else in common except for the daily ritual of tea. Tea, the inhabitants of these very different countries say, warms you when you are feeling cold, cools you when you are hot, calms you when you are agitated and lifts you up when you are feeling down. A cup of tea means a moment of quiet and peace; as one sips a sense of 'ahness' pervades the mind, the body and the spirit as a state of grace seems to descend upon us. The ritual of tea can be seen as a very modest and small form of spiritual retreat: we are being there, quietly doing nothing except contemplating, in the goodness of the moment. These simple pleasures are where we cultivate the sense of the sacred every day.

Spirituality is seeded, germinates, sprouts and blossoms in our kitchens too. The kitchen has been regarded throughout history as a place of enchantment: this is where the hearth and the heart of the house are. In fact, kitchens help us transform a house into a home. More problems are solved and joys celebrated here than in any other part of the house. It is in the kitchen where we become alchemists every day and transform, like Babette in the tale, raw ingredients into food for the soul. It is also a place for meditation. As we cut vegetables, peel potatoes, choose what foods to cook, or watch water come to a boil, we gain a taste of silence and 'of being in the moment'. The enchantment is also to be found in all the kitchen utensils we use for cooking and it is nurtured in the way we prepare meals. We all have favourite pots that cook better than any other, no matter how old or battered they are; or certain peelers, knives or glasses which hold a special kind of magic that works again and again. Paying attention to the magic that is at work in the kitchen is an art – cooking soulfully – which may be enriched by the memory of a past when food was indeed sacred.

The first altar of mankind was the primitive hearth, a white mound of tightly packed ashes which kept the fire from dying. This is where the tribe gathered, seeking sanctuary from a world of darkness and predators, to weave tales of hunting exploits and to honour their guardian spirits. The white of the ashes was maintained as the colour of temples throughout antiquity and it came to be associated with purity. Interestingly, many of our modern kitchens are still white today. If we lift the veils of history to uncover how our ancestors regarded food, we may be surprised to learn that although time has passed, some aspects of life have been maintained.

THE PREHISTORIC DIET

The connection between food and religion is extremely ancient, dating back to when the early Indo-European nomadic tribes came to settle, over centuries, in small communities and turned from violent hunters into more peace-loving gatherers. The need to grow food, rather than hunt for it, marked the beginning of civilisation as the agrarian lifestyle fostered stability in population growth, technological advancement and social complexity. Religious art, ritual objects, carvings and archaeological remains dating from that period help us define the image of existence as it was then: life-sustaining, nature-worshipping communities of men and women whose intimate relationship with the earth was paramount to their survival.

Far and wide in the geography of the sacred, we find temples, sanctuaries and other religious structures erected as early as the Neolithic period to map the movements of the sun and moon and their influence upon the crops. Ancient places such as Stonehenge and Avebury in England are important psychic records of a time when people – lacking our scientific knowledge but possessing powerful mystical intuition and wisdom – tried to explain, study and influence the cycles of nature. Their survival depended almost exclusively upon successful harvests, and this vital bond created a mystical participation with the earth from which their daily food was derived. There are many religious myths, spanning a huge period of time and landscape, that explicitly place agriculture and farming as the hallowed bond between the divine and mankind: food is life and thus it is sacred. Food was offered to the gods upon these ancient altars; it was placed within burial sites to sustain the departed in their journey to the other world. The need to find fertile plains determined where the greatest civilisations flowered.

Primitive cities acquired power by being able to store food and prevent potential threats such as famine, disease and marauding tribes from annihilating them. The storage of food in Egypt and ancient Babylon was presided over by priests who also studied the movements of the sun and moon and were able to make accurate predictions on the outcome of forthcoming harvests. Syrius, the star thought to influence the waters of the Nile, was worshipped as a divinity as its visibility in the sky at a certain time of the year marked the flooding of the great river which made the fields of Egypt fertile and guaranteed the survival of the land of Pharaohs.

The great urban civilisations of Mesopotamia – Babylon, Sumer and Assyria – which developed in Asia Minor nearly 5,000 years ago and the reputedly even more ancient settlements of Old Europe have left us with a legacy that is relevant to us today: the primitive diet. It mainly consisted of grains – wheat, barley, corn, millet – which were regarded as sacred gifts from Mother Earth, farmed vegetables and pulses. This simple but nourishing diet has been the staple of mankind for millennia; it included little meat as most proteins and other nutrients are contained in grains and pulses. This stable combination was sustained throughout history; the universal commonality of the grinding stones found amidst archaeological remains of prehistoric villages shows us that grains formed the basis of all meals in the past. From the Celts to the Aztecs, from the ancient Egyptians to the classical Greeks, from the native Americans to the African tribes – everyone grew, harvested, ground and cooked grains every day of their lives. The maintenance of a grain-based diet is further supported by the first written history of our own culture: Rome survived on its wheat and barley, on which even the conquering legions were fed. Medieval annals report that people throughout Europe ate mostly grains and some vegetables; ancient monastery records from France, Italy and Germany again inform us that grains, wild herbs and vegetables appeared at the refectory table. North Italian dishes such as risotto, polenta, pasta e fagioli, which are very fashionable today, formed the grain-based winter diet of farmers and peasants for many centuries as the ingredients were both cheap and warmth-inducing. The thought that the race of mankind has been sustained on this diet for nearly 7,000 years is staggering. Today, the people of Asia are still nourished by the daily bowl of rice.

Joseph Campbell, in his authoritative study of the world's mythologies, *The Masks of God*, states that the two different attitudes towards life and death, the corner-stones of human existence, are essentially dietary. People whose nutrition is based upon the fruits of the earth have over millennia come to feel a deep bond and respect for nature and they view human existence as non-violent and following the same cycle as plants: birth, life, death and rebirth. This attitude is now predominantly Eastern, as Asian people are mostly vegetarian and have a deep faith in this 'eternal return' which is mirrored in their religion and mythology. People who kill in order to eat regard existence as being essentially brutal and violent: birth, life and death, which is inevitably followed by the punishment of hell or eternal torment inflicted by vindictive ghosts and spirits. This view has been the prerogative of the West and is reflected in its monotheistic religions – Christianity, Judaism and Islam – which are based upon the struggle between good and evil and which do not believe in the concept of the reincarnation of the soul.

It is this long-established habit of eating grains, pulses and vegetables which makes it the ideal diet for our bodies; our digestive systems have been shaped on this staple for many thousands of years. Macrobiotic, Ayurvedic, Chinese and other methods of healing by use of certain foods are based upon this diet. If in the West we have departed from this way of eating, it is only because the abundance of 'fast foods' and ready-made meals has progressively confused our instinct about nutrition over the last three decades. Technology, while gifting us with plenty, has also contributed to the abstraction of the idea of food; as we no longer cultivate what we eat, it removes us further and further away from the original source of food. We now read on the back of packaging about its provenance and its chemical components. Baking our own bread is an entirely different experience than buying it already sliced and shrink-wrapped in an anonymous counter at a superstore. When we return to the original way of eating, something happens to our interiority; we suddenly discover the soul of food that emerges when we cook with the basic ingredients which have been used for thousands of years.

Today, when we visit Thai, Japanese, Indian or Chinese restaurants we not only gain an experience of a different way of eating, but we also return to the essential and most healthy diet for our bodies. Asian countries, financially less affluent than our own, have maintained this ancient way of eating because the average household can afford to feed many on grains, pulses and vegetables; meat, fish and sweets are still luxuries to be eaten only on special occasions. A number of modern diseases and health afflictions such as allergies, candida yeast infections, diabetes, digestive disorders, heart disease, low and high blood pressure, hyperactivity in children and many types of cancer have been proven to be both prevented and cured by this form of diet.

Of all ways of eating, this is the most spiritual diet for mankind; it is ancient and it balances mind, body and soul in a way that no other food combination does. This is the diet still followed today in monasteries, temples, and retreat centres – modern day sanctuaries to heal us both from within and without. Many participants of weekend retreats at Tassajara, the successful Buddhist monastery in California, say that the regeneration they feel at soul level is as much due to the food served at mealtimes as the spiritual exercises they undertake. Tassajara offers a simple but rich vegetarian cuisine of organic produce; a variety of vegetables, grains and pulses form the basis of every meal. This formula proved to be so successful that the monastery opened what is now a thriving restaurant in San Francisco where people can have a taste of Buddhist fare California-style any time.

ZEN FOOD

Handle even a single leaf of a green in such a way that it manifests the body of the Buddha. This in turn allows the Buddha to manifest through the leaf. This is a power which you cannot grasp with your rational mind. It operates freely, according to the situation, in a most natural way. At the same time, this power functions in our lives to clarify and settle activities and is beneficial to all living things.
– Zen Master Eihei Dogen Zenji, *From the Zen Kitchen to Enlightenment*

The beauty of the Zen monasteries that dot the Japanese rural landscape is as much due to the natural forests and bamboo groves which guard their privacy as to the quality of meditation that pervades their every corner. Perfectly tended gardens, gravel raked in undulating formations adorning the passageways, black meditation cushions carefully arranged in the *Zendo* (meditation hall) where the sound of raindrops upon the garden rocks deepen the experience of *zazen* (sitting silently in the lotus position): the outside has been modelled to mirror the inner enlightenment cultivated daily by Zen monks and nuns. One of the most essential functions in a Zen monastery is that of chief cook, or *tenzo* in Japanese. From ancient times this work has been carried out by teachers well versed in the Buddha's Way and who have aroused the *bodhisattva* spirit (the ability to bring enlightenment upon others) within them. The duty of the *tenzo* is to prepare the community's meals and to care for the physical and spiritual well-being of its members so as to '...enable everyone to practise with their bodies and minds with the least hindrance'. This is how Zen Master Eihei Dogen Zenji (1200–1253) wrote in his book *From the Zen Kitchen to Enlightenment* which is still regarded today as a unique guide to how we should go about cooking in a spiritual, wholesome and enlightened way. He wrote the treatise because he was saddened that, although the Buddha's Way had been introduced in Japan for several hundred years, no-one had ever written about the preparation and serving of meals as an expression of *buddhadharma* (Buddha's Law). It is the *tenzo*'s ability to see the soul in food and to cook soulfully for his fellow travellers that makes his office so important to the whole community. This regard

can be a lesson for our own households: let us remember to thank and honour our own *tenzos* for taking care of us. We don't think twice about thanking a restaurant chef, and yet at home we often fall into disputes because of this simple negligence as so many home cooks feel their efforts are forever being taken for granted!

Zen is the practice of awareness in everything in every moment; although *zazen* is a fundamental application of the Zen Way, meditation is brought to many other activities: gardening, cooking, eating, walking, cleaning and being. This attitude underscores a spiritual urgency: 'Wake up now!' is the inherent message to everything Zen. Eating thus becomes an exercise in enlightenment and Zen monasteries have their own unique table manners. The period before the meals is always dedicated to meditation and the silence is carried on to the table where speaking is forbidden. This may remind us of those horrible silences imposed upon the family by thundering fathers and grandfathers who professed that 'not talking at the table is a sign of good manners'! Eating silently, however, can be a very soulful experience. Many of us are forced into eating alone at the office when there are just not enough hours in the day to complete all of our tasks, and going out to a restaurant becomes a time-consuming luxury that cannot be afforded. In these moments we not only save time, but we can also practise eating Zen-style.

EATING ALONE

Close the door to your office or choose a space where you can be alone. Relax for two or three minutes by paying attention to the in and out of your breathing. You may feel like keeping your eyes closed to disengage from computer screens or activities of the mind. Now, unwrap your food and lay it out aesthetically before you; everything must be there – drink, napkin, cutlery – so that you don't have to interrupt your silence in the middle of your eating alone meditation. Eat slowly, chew carefully, savour each ingredient and feel the goodness of it. Swallow each bite before putting the next one in. Be total in your eating alone, don't look at work documents, magazines or other distractions; pay attention to what you are eating. This silence will make your eating graceful and elegant. Drink slowly and only after having swallowed each bite. Look at the way the body responds when it is being nourished. Slow your breathing pattern and allow satisfaction to expand the experience. Pause when switching from one course to the next; allow the body to adjust to the different textures and flavours. When you finish, again close your eyes, pay attention to your breathing and be grateful for the abundance you have received.

Zen monks and nuns silently recite *sutras* before and after each meal. This is the equivalent of the prayer-before-the-meal practice of Christian households. Prayers and recitation of *sutras* are intended as an honouring of the soul of food and awaken awareness of what we are about to do. They also bring us a few moments of silence and quiet contemplation; disengaging from the activities of the day, we pause before taking nourishment into our bodies. These are some popular Zen meal *sutras*:

• Considering the meal's effect, we reflect on whence it came
• Weighing our virtues, we accept this offering
• To defend against our delusive minds and separate ourselves from our faults, we must first of all overcome greed
• To cure our bodily weakness, we take this fine medicine
• To attain enlightenment, we now eat this food

So little thought goes to the elements that bring food onto our table: sunshine, rain, fertile soil and the people who pick and package it for us. The first *sutra* draws our attention to where the food came from that is necessary in order to appreciate its goodness. All food is an offering of the Earth and we as its children partake in its bounty; the second *sutra* reminds us that the Earth goes on producing our food no matter what injury we inflict upon its lands, seas, trees and animals. The planet is far kinder to us than we are proving to be to it. Greed, the subject of the third *sutra,* is that which prevents us from sharing food equally. The Third World's hand-to-mouth is the Westerner's abundance and although this may seem a painful and unpleasant reminder, this imbalance will not be corrected until it is fully realised by each one of us individually and collectively. The fourth *sutra* teaches us that in order to maintain excellent health we need to treat food as medicine. We have largely forgotten the healing properties of meals, but this instinct can be reawakened as we pay closer attention to how our body responds to what we eat. The last *sutra* is an encouragement to attain enlightenment even in the simple act of eating: when we align mind, body and spirit and focus totally on the action in the moment we are in *satori* (Zen enlightenment). Master Shunryu Suzuki Roshi ends his book *Zen Mind, Beginner's Mind* with the sentence 'In

Japan in the spring we eat cucumbers' — this is it, he is saying; spiritual wholeness does not need to be grand and other-worldly; it is the very simple act of being here, on a spring day eating cucumbers.

Zen meals are based on the primitive staple of grains, vegetables and pulses forming a delicious and nutritious vege-tarian diet. In fact, most temples and monasteries follow this same diet the world over — throughout the Buddhist countries of South-east Asia, in Taoist China; even some Roman Catholic monas-teries have adopted mostly vegetarian fare. Zen monasteries include in their meals all seasonal vegetables as well as herbs that grow in the surrounding fields, forests and riverbanks, such as some mountain grass and tree leaves, horsetail, starwort, dande-lion, sorrel, wild butterbur, sprouts, wisteria buds, parsley, trefoil, red beans, gingko nuts and lily bulbs. These ingredi-ents are combined with wholemeal rice and various beans to form a meal which is high in nutrients, proteins and vitamins. The monastic diet coupled with medita-tion has been demonstrated to be the winning formula for the most advanced stress-reduction techniques used in the West today. Applying ancient methods to modern day malaises such as chronic stress, mental fatigue and heart disease is proving not only one of the most valid preventative methods, but also a system to which patients are responding positively in terms of both health improvements and personal fulfilment.

MEDITATION AND DIET

Simply meditate every day before you take food. Close your eyes and just feel what your body needs. . .You have not seen any food. . . you are simply feeling your own being, what your body needs, what you feel like, what you hanker for. . . This [is] 'humming food' — food that hums to you. Go and eat as much of it as you want, but stick to it. The other food [is called] 'beckoning food': when it becomes available, you become interested in it. Then it is a mind thing and it is not your need. If you listen to your humming food, you can eat as much as you want and you will never suffer, because it will satisfy you. The body simply desires that which it needs; it never desires anything else. That will be satisfactory, and once there is satisfaction, one never eats more. The problem arises only if you are eating foods which are beckoning foods: you see them avail-able and you become interested and you eat. They cannot satisfy you because there is no need in the body for them. When they don't satisfy you, you feel unsatisfied. Feeling unsatisfied, you eat more . . . it is not going to satisfy you because there is no need in the body in the first place.

— Osho, *From Medication to Meditation*

The great contemporary master Osho tells us about an ancient yogic saying that states that the food which is best is the one that 'hums' to you; ordinary food, by con-trast, does not emit a low resonance — we are visually or mentally attracted to it, but when ingested we may feel it was the wrong kind of meal. Chicken soup is the cliché feel-good food for Jews, food that 'hums' and makes us feel spiritually better after eating it. In India, the land that gave rise to meditation, ancient masters used to teach their disciples that the first temple is the body. We should worship the body, pay attention and care for it, so that the soul within us can shine outwards. Food is the first and most basic substance for our health as it heals us from sickness, it strengthens us and ensures that we stay healthy. The type and quality of the food we eat, and how it is consumed is determined by our degree of awareness of our body – the more sensitive, the more perceptive we are, the greater the attention for what we eat. Normally, however, unless we are suffering from a weight or general health disorder, we tend to consume food which we relish – we are attracted to it visually and become hungry for it because of the anticipated pleasure it will give us in our palate. But do we know whether or not it is good for us? Do we know whether it will cause stress or relieve it; whether it will increase our energy or slow us down? Most probably not.

The neglect over our diet affects us immediately and seriously – we may be over or underweight, we may be obsessive about food, we may seriously suffer from lack of energy or be afflicted by a yo-yo dynamism which roller-coasters us from peaks to valleys within a twelve-hour cycle. Our temptation is not to relate the activities that go on in our bodies and minds with the kind of food we eat. But if we consider that the *only* and basic reason why we eat at all is to keep us fuelled, then the connection becomes crystal clear. We wouldn't dream of injecting low-quality fuel into our cars, so why would we not pay attention to what kind of food we eat? Some of us may be shocked to discover that we know the mechanisms of our cars and personal computers better than the inner workings of our body.

The role of diets in health and health disorders has been studied for years, and we now know that diet affects our health very quickly. For instance, even a single meal high in fat and cholesterol may induce the body to release a hormone called *thromboxane* which causes the arteries to constrict and the blood to clot faster. That is why heart patients get chest pains after eating a fatty meal, and why so many of them end up in the emergency ward after a rich Christmas or Thanksgiving feast.

We also know that the role of moderate but regular physical activity is vital in maintaining a healthy metabolism – exercise is the second component of the health equation. Studies over the last two decades have proven that stress is the third crucial element for our health. There are two kinds: acute and chronic. We are designed to cope with acute stress far better than with chronic stress, and yet if we stop and examine our modern existence, we would have to admit most of us meet stress on a daily, if not hourly, basis, and thus are frighteningly familiar with the term chronic stress as being a constant in our lives.

Recent pioneering and revolutionary studies by, among others, Dr. Dean Ornish, President and Director of the Preventive Medicine Research Institute in Sausalito (California), and by Dr. Jon Kabat-Zinn, founder and Director of the Stress Reduction Clinic at the University of Massachusetts Medical Center, have scientifically proven that meditation and diet are both extremely important key factors in our health. Their studies have provided the missing link in the chain of causes and effects that keep us healthy – meditation addresses our spiritual well-being. The immediate effect of meditation is to make us more conscious of the way we are and thus help us change all those patterns that are harmful to us. Diet and exercise make our body fit and sound, stress reduction keeps our mind alert, and meditation awakens our spirit to the beauty and wonder of each moment. Meditation is now considered equal in importance to the other three factors in maintaining our well-being, and no modern healthcare programme is considered complete unless it includes elements of meditation.

Meditation is the art of paying attention, of creating a state in which we are simply silent yet fully alert and, in its deepest state, meditation is the absence of thoughts and the full presence of awareness. This is an ongoing process, an awakened alertness to every action: when we breathe, how we breathe; when we walk, how we walk; when we eat, how we eat. When one is paying attention there is a subtle but powerful shift of perception. Suddenly we watch ourselves as though from a distance, and we become less gripped by exterior stimuli – without, however, losing any concentration on our daily tasks. When this shift occurs we cannot help but be more conscious of how we do things; our concentration increases because we are able to focus more fully upon each moment. The natural consequence of meditation is that we start to care for our bodies, ourselves and others too. Rather than withdrawing from the world, meditation can help us enjoy it more fully, more effectively and more peacefully. It brings an increased appreciation to how we feel – we become progressively more sensitive to what is good for us and thus more discerning about how we conduct our lives. The Buddhists call this increased perception 'mindfulness' and consider it to be the heart of Buddhist teaching.

Modern medical research and ancient temple techniques are now being combined to re-educate our instincts about how we lead our lives. Many patients who were suffering from severe heart conditions have been healed by adopting a grain-based vegetarian diet – the primitive diet – with meditation. Correct eating is fundamental to our health not only when we are sick, but also if we are intent on keeping our well-being, vitality and wish to lead longer, happier lives.

Our natural instinct for food is as a silent, slow and almost secluded act, very far from the noisy activities of a busy lunchtime restaurant or the quick-grabbing of a sandwich from a street corner vendor. Seeing a small baby suckling from its mother's breast is an awe-inspiring experience. Both mother and baby are silent and we naturally feel a reverence to this act; we feel like intruders who should not watch, for it is something private and bond-forming between the two of them. Dinners with our families and friends can sometimes feel like a blessing and a celebration to our souls – it is not just mere consumption of food, it is an honouring of life at a deep level. In the past, families used to sit around the table and pray before starting their meal. Prayers before food are a common expression of devotion in many religions. People not only thank their gods for the food served, but they also stop for a moment of silence, breaking away in their thoughts from daily activities and reaching a different level of awareness before eating. Throughout the East it is considered unclean to eat unless one has washed. On arriving home in the evening, for instance, all Japanese people take a bath before the meal, soaking in clean water, resting and soothing tired limbs, joints and brains. After the bath they wear a *yukata*, a simple cotton house robe. Clean, warm, comfortable, refreshed and relaxed, they can now begin the evening meal.

> *There is rice in my bag*
> *For ten days,*
> *And a bundle of firewood*
> *By the hearth.*
>
> – Ryokan

Modern life has divorced us completely from our natural instincts about food. When we buy it in supermarkets, for instance, we are bombarded by so many stimuli that appeal to the outer senses that our inner sense is completely drowned. By contrast, we all remember the great pleasure and satisfaction of spring and summer days spent planting and picking vegetables and fruit from our gardens, or the pride we feel when we bring back some special food from a countryside outing: freshly picked strawberries from the field, home-made wine, or natural raw honey. These items possess greater value than their supermarket equivalents because we know that there are human hands behind their making and packaging. Someone has been in the field to pick fruit for us; someone else has dressed up in an bee-keeper's suit to gather the honey. We know of someone who even takes his bees on holidays, packing them on the back of an old van, so that they may enjoy different flowers in different fields and thus produce a greater variety of honey. These are people who care about the product and that care is transmitted to us. They have paid attention and may even have been in a state of silent meditation as they did their work – what they do, how they do it is the goodness we buy. Meditation is not just merely sitting silently in the lotus pose; meditation is about care, appreciation, the heart and soul of life and everything we are and do in it.

Chapter 2

The Diet for a New Humanity

When washing the rice, remove any sand you find. In doing so, do not lose even one grain of rice. When you look at the rice see the sand at the same time; when you look at the sand see also the rice. Examine both carefully. Then, a meal containing the six flavours and the three qualities will come together naturally.

– Zen Master Eihei Dogen Zenji, *From the Zen Kitchen to Enlightenment*

Zen Master Eihei Dogen Zenji uses 'rice' and 'sand' both literally and metaphorically; rice represents enlightenment and sand represents illusion, the two polarities of the spiritual path. All life flows between two opposite poles: dark and light, heaven and earth, male and female, hot and cold, good and bad, matter and spirit. Everything we can think of contains elements of both as nothing is just either one or the other. This is a principle that was well understood by the Chinese theory of *yin* and *yang* which states that all objects and phenomena in the universe can be seen as limitless pairs of opposites; the source of *yin* and *yang* is the ultimate balance, that which is eternal. The *yin–yang* symbol shows a circle formed by two fish – one white and one black; the white fish has a dark eye and the black fish has a white eye, thus creating a completely balanced picture. The *yin* principle is

everything shadowy, cool, dark and feminine; it is believed that this power commences in the autumn, overcoming the sun and giving way to the coldness and darkness of winter. The *yang* principle is the opposite, representing everything that is hot, light and expansive. *Yang* power commences in the spring, waking the world from the sleep of winter and making nature grow its bounty through the summer. We have naturally applied this ancient Chinese principle to our own lives and diets: in cold climates (*yin*), we eat warm foods (*yang*) and vice versa. When we feel hot (*yang*), we consume more fluids (*yin*); when we are greatly active (*yang*), we need periods of rest (*yin*). Respecting the law of polar opposites brings us balance, health, well-being and joy.

The *yin–yang* principle gives us a very easy method for balancing our diets according to our own personal needs at any one point in time. All foods, both solids and liquids, can be divided into essentially *yin* or essentially *yang* and in order to maintain health we need a combination of both. Our immediate environment also contains elements of *yin* and *yang*; a stressful, aggressive office is overly yang; our favourite armchair at home, placed in a peaceful, secluded room is *yin*. Activities follow the same principle, with working weekdays being *yang* and relaxed weekends spent with family and friends being *yin*. Once we become accustomed to viewing these qualities both within ourselves, in what we do and in the world that surrounds us, we can easily monitor our diets to obtain the maximum potential and benefits. If we are stressed at work, we will eat *yin* food to ease the tension and achieve clarity and focus. If we are suffering from a winter cold, with fevers and shivers, we will be naturally drawn to *yang* food to replenish our physical energy and to keep us warm. Our own internal harmony depends upon the balancing of *yin* and *yang*: when we have equal amounts of both in our bodies we experience harmony as good health and well-being.

We suggest that you cut out or copy the *yin–yang* charts for food and cooking methods and keep them in your kitchen, so that you can refer to them whenever you are about to start preparing your meals. Start experimenting with the *yin–yang* correspondences between the foods you eat and the way you are feeling at any one point in time. Learn by paying attention to your body, mind and soul.

Food can either increase or decrease our daily stress levels. Opposite we give you a learn-at-a-glance guide to the stress levels caused by certain foods. Again, we suggest that you cut out or copy this chart and keep it handy at the office or in your kitchen. You may want to refer to it when going out to a restaurant at lunch-time, when ordering take-away food or when you are so stressed you'd do anything to get some peace and quiet!

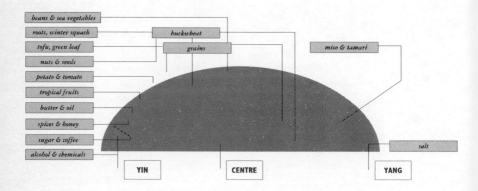

beans & sea vegetables
roots, winter squash
tofu, green leaf
nuts & seeds
potato & tomato
tropical fruits
butter & oil
spices & honey
sugar & coffee
alcohol & chemicals

buckwheat
grains

miso & tamari

salt

YIN   CENTRE   YANG

FOODS WHICH INCREASE STRESS LEVELS	FOODS WHICH DECREASE STRESS LEVELS
Eggs	Tofu
Meat	Tempeh
Fried food	Pinto, lima and soy beans
Cheese	Oatmeal
Salmon	Soy products
Cream	Goat's milk
Whole milk	Tahini
Butter	Unrefined oils
Mayonnaise	Sesame, sunflower and pumpkin seeds
Nuts	Corn tortillas
Palm and coconut oils	Muesli
Avocados	Pies with low oil crust
Fried chips	RiceDream
Cookies and cakes of all types	Salads
Pizza	Fresh yoghurt

You can prepare some of these items ahead of time and keep them handy in the refrigerator, either at home or in the office. For instance, tahini or toasted sunflower seeds (which can be kept in a plastic storage box) make wonderful toppings on rice cakes when you get a craving. Try to observe the moments when you feel like grabbing for food because you are feeling stressed; invariably you will feel like eating something sweet. Sugar gives you a temporary high, followed by a low, which you may adjust with yet more sugar. Let craving-watching be your office meditation and find healthier alternatives. Keep instant miso soup packets and corn tortillas with a delicious dip by your desk for one day and notice the difference when you eat these things rather than sugar – you will eat less and be more satisfied.

Applying the *yin–yang* principle is not a matter of learning something entirely new; this ancient wisdom recalls our own instinct about what is right for us at any one point in time. Paying attention, being sensitive to how we feel and what we need, approaching life in a meditative way, seeking balance and harmony in our emotions, actions and relationships – these are the tools we all possess and that enable us to apply wisdom and enlightenment to our lives. Rather than absorbing yet another dietary system, the *yin–yang* principle awakens our natural instinct about correct eating – we will choose 'humming' food, substances we need rather than crave.

THE MODERN DIET

Let him extend unboundedly
His heart to every living thing.
Buddha

Today we benefit from an abundance of knowledge, technology and skills in growing the highest quality food, yet we suffer from diverse dietary ailments. For the first time in United States history, the Surgeon General acknowledged in 1988 the value of a good diet as reportedly two-thirds of all deaths are directly affected by improper diets. Poor eating habits play a large part in the nation's most common killers – coronary heart disease, stroke, atherosclerosis, diabetes and some cancers. What we need now is an intelligent diet – we need to function at the peak of our energies and to maintain that balance with a minimum of upkeep. Food can act as foundation medicine. If diet is used correctly, we will be less prone to life-damaging illnesses and require less medicine.

This era will one day in the future be known as the convergence between East and West, and this fundamental meeting is mirrored in the way we eat as much as in many other areas of life. Our supermarkets now stock exotic fruit and vegetables as well as sea vegetables, wholegrain breads and pastas, with staples from Indian, Japanese and Chinese culinary traditions. Seeing the different produce on the shelves is an open invitation to customers to experiment with other methods of cooking and eating. Innumerable television and radio programmes teach us endlessly how to prepare meals that originated in far and away parts of the world. These are everyday manifestations of an integration of oriental food medicine and occidental nutrition. Thousands of years ago, master healers in the Orient devised simple yet incredibly effective methods of healing their patients with food. Analysing the human being as a total composite of body, mind and soul, they created a fully comprehensive spectrum of guidelines about diet as the first and foremost cure for all common ailments. Oriental medicine

offers a different dimension of food from our own. It recognises the warming and cooling values of certain ingredients, the ability to moisten, strengthen energy, calm the mind, reduce watery or mucoid accumulations, and many other imbalances of the mind, the body and the spirit. Western nutrition can benefit enormously from the ancient wisdom of the East – while we speak of carbohydrates, proteins and fats, we can also learn from cleansing, de-stressing and enlightening foods. The modern diet is the perfect marriage of these two great traditions and the recipes in this book are based upon the most recent discoveries of both areas.

As the affluent West becomes progressively more interested in a holistic approach to the body and to life, so we become interested in incorporating ancient oriental wisdom into our homes. We may combine exercise with meditation, and a rich joyful diet with those nutrient qualities that enhance our health. This is a sign that we are paying attention, bringing ancient temple techniques into our offices and homes, and that we care not only about our bodies but also our souls. We are now aware of soul quality in our lives more than in the recent past and we are making efforts to increase its presence in everything.

The best foods to use for long-term balance of body, mind and spirit are not extreme; they are mild and centring and form an axis around which other, more extreme, ingredients can revolve (see Summary of Basic Nutrients chart on page 24). These mild ingredients are the complex carbohydrates found in the original diets the world over and the staples of the primitive diet discussed in the previous chapter. This large group contains grains, vegetables, sea vegetables, legumes, nuts and seeds and fruit – now popularly recognised under the modern term fibre. Complex carbohydrates contain the most balanced amounts of *yin* and *yang* energy; they increase, build and maintain harmony both within our bodies and between us and the environment. The race of mankind has eaten combinations of these ingredients for millennia and they still represent the most intelligent way of eating today. The recipes in this book revolve around the intelligent use of complex carbohydrates for maximum health and nutrition. Readers will find that the meals are delicious, easily digested and produce large amounts of energy which allow us to work at the peak of our energies without having to snack between meals. Complex carbohydrates also accomplish another, perhaps more magical function: when our diets are based on them, we feel more peaceful, more alert and naturally more soulful. This is because we have drastically reduced the amount of toxic substances that cause havoc in our digestive systems and which keep the vital organs, such as the liver, working overtime to re-establish the balance that is lost by our way of eating. When our bodies are nourished with a healthy, clean diet something happens to the rest of us. Our energy channels clear, our ability to focus increases, our weight returns to a normal level, we are less prone to sickness and, unburdened by poisons and toxins, we feel happier and naturally closer in spirit to the rest of life.

A VEGETARIAN DIET

The modern diet is ultimately a vegetarian one based upon the extensive and expert use of complex carbohydrates. The recipes in this book follow a vegetarian way of nutrition and have been carefully devised for maximum vitality and variety in their presentation. Food for the soul does not require the taking of animal life; we need to take from the exterior that which is going to give our interior vital energy, and this does not include the act of killing. Food for the soul demands that we recognise soul quality not only in ourselves, our homes and relationships, but also in the world that surrounds us, in the animals and plants. We very seldom see the way domestic animals are bred, fed and killed before they reach our tables; images of this process deeply affect our human sensitivity. The debate over the British problem of BSE (mad cow disease) alerted a large proportion of the public to the fact that the quality of animal life and health was sacrificed in order to satisfy our demand for beef. As soon as short documentary images of diseased cows, of the contents of their feed (protein derived from, among other things, sheep's entrails) and their inevitable destiny at the slaughterhouse reached our homes, many of us felt that this was a very cruel and unnatural way of treating farm animals. Shopping in supermarkets, although very convenient, ultimately robs us of the direct experience of the origins of food. If we really *knew* and *saw* the ingredients of tinned food, the farms where the animals are kept, the fields where our grains are harvested, we would have an entirely different approach to shopping. Even the act of thinking about these issues already changes our perception of nutrition. When we begin to think in terms of energy forces – the energy of something which is outside being introduced into our own interiority – then our sensitivity to food and the way we prepare our meals increases a thousandfold.

Many people are under the impression that the absence of meat in the diet leads to a grave protein deficiency. However, when certain vegetables, pulses and grains are combined intelligently they offer better quality protein than meat. Toxins in plants and grains are far fewer than in meat and are readily neutralised in the process of cooking. In order to be preserved, meat needs to be treated with nitrate (a toxic substance for us), which is released at different cooking temperatures. When meat toxins are introduced into the acidic climate of our stomach they create serious internal disarray – so our stomachs need to work harder to digest meat.

The recipes in this book also make minimal use of dairy food and eggs, two of the most prevalent allergens today. We are so used to including these ingredients in our meals that we have no experience of what would happen to our bodies if we were to eliminate them for a while or dramatically decrease their use in our daily food. The meals are an invitation to try and see what happens; those suffering from skin or respiratory allergies will notice a remarkable difference in a very short time. Those people who are not affected by allergies will also recognise the benefits of a dairy-free diet: their weight will drop and they will generally feel less obstructed and gain more energy.

Vegetarianism does not lead to enlightenment. Jesus ate meat and completely transformed centuries of spiritual thinking, and so too, many others like him. However, the increased awareness that comes from meditation, from caring for ourselves and others, does dramatically alter the way we feel about the world. Meditation renews the bond between the individual and the universe that surrounds us and this includes the animal kingdom. It is very difficult to dig your knife and fork into a carcass that has been fried and call it a good meal when you are in a state of increased sensitivity and perception. Meditation also alters our appreciation of aesthetics – spirituality goes hand in hand with beauty; when this is applied to our diet, it is simple to see how the sense of aesthetics can be enhanced far more with vegetables and grains than with dead animals.

In oriental countries, rich in their tradition of spirituality and meditation, even the ordinary householder follows rules of asceticism. The whole of Hindu society, for instance, cultivates the ideal of *ahimsa,* or non-injury. This is the absence of the desire to harm, manifested in the Hindu preference for a vegetarian diet and in the worship of the cow, an animal which gives food without needing to be killed. In the East, most people know that eating food which is pure leads to a purity in the physical, mental and spiritual eco-system.

ORGANIC FOOD

The Earth does not belong to us. We belong to the Earth.
– Chief Seattle, of the Suqwamish and Duwamish, an ally of the white man and a key figure in the agreement to settle the Washington tribes in reservations in 1855.

The vitality gained with food for the soul is also based upon the attention and respect we give to the preparation of our meals. When we care for the soul of the ingredients we are chopping, slicing, boiling and laying out on serving dishes, the quality of the meal is enhanced. Our attention creates a certain atmosphere around the table and this can be applied not only to our family dinners, but also on those occasions when we invite friends. The success of dinner parties is in the combination of the right people – the right atmosphere is created by the hosts and the guests feel cared for and happy. The more we pay heed to atmosphere and to the quality of certain moments, the more these are revealed to us. It is like looking into a divining well and seeing patterns and shapes; the more we look, the more we can read the secrets and revelations in the water.

Finding soul in food also leads us to greater awareness of the kind of food we buy. Today, most cities and country villages have a few stores or supermarkets which specialise in organic food or have a section dedicated to organic produce. In its original sense, all food is organic because it comes from plants or animals. However, in the last fifty years or so, the term organic has been used to describe food grown without fertilisers or pesticides and in a way that emphasises crop rotation, so as to ensure that the life of the soil has been maintained. Organic fruit and vegetables have been grown in a traditional, environmentally-friendly way. Organic farmers follow organic production systems which are designed to produce optimum quantities of food of high nutritional quality by using management practices which minimise damage to the environment and wildlife. These include: working with natural systems rather than seeking to dominate them; the encouragement of biological cycles involving micro-organisms, soil flora and fauna, plants and animals; the maintenance of valuable existing landscape features and adequate habitats for the production of wildlife with particular regard to endangered species; careful attention to

animal welfare; the avoidance of pollution; and consideration for the wider social and ecological impact of the farming system. A great deal of care, soul and attention goes into organic farming and as a consequence the products are more expensive than the average fruit and vegetables that may have been sprayed with harmful pesticides and grown with chemical fertilisers. The trend, however, is that the public is increasingly demanding that such products be sold in ordinary supermarkets and that an extensive range of health foods be offered on their counters. The more we care about the soul, the more discerning we become about the environment and how to treat it. In the near future we will hopefully see a greater abundance of organic produce in our shops, selling at more affordable prices. We encourage you to include organic fruit and vegetables in your meals; also produce which is in season and grown locally is generally not more expensive than non-organically cultivated food. The difference, however, is remarkable: it tastes better and is more fulfilling. You will also want to eat comparatively less organic produce as all the original vitality has been preserved in the fruit and vegetables – less satisfies more.

LIVING IN HARMONY WITH THE SEASONS: THE CHINESE FIVE ELEMENT THEORY

The Five Element theory was developed thousands of years ago by Chinese sages who saw the limitless correspondences between the workings of the human body and the workings of nature. It is a simple and yet effective way of describing the constitution and condition of any individual at any one point in the year. The five elements – wood, fire, earth, metal and water – correspond to five seasons – spring, midsummer, late summer, autumn and winter. Between these two parameters there exist other sets of correspondences between the inside of our bodies and the environment. Each element and season also relate to a physical organ, to a taste, to a degree of *yin–yang* balance and to certain foods which help us attune to the seasons.

The Five Element theory is a workable model that allows us to see all the natural correspondences and how we are affected by them. The elements, and everything that relates to them, influence one another either positively – forming a creative cycle – or negatively – forming a destructive cycle. The creation cycle can briefly be explained as:

Wood burns to make
Fire whose ashes decompose into
Earth where they are born and mined as
Metals which enrich
Water which nourishes trees (*wood*)

The destruction cycle is explained as:

Wood is cut by *Metal*
Fire is extinguished by *Water*
Earth is penetrated by *Wood*
Metal is melted by *Fire*
Water is channelled and contained by
Earth

Our internal organs release either positive or negative energy in the measure that they are affected by the changes in the environment. We all know that we need to brace ourselves against a very cold day with layers of warm clothes, hot stews and stimulating beverages. However, we might feel that spring is a very disorienting season, taking us through highs and lows of energy, affecting our heads and our general re-energising potential. Each change of season causes a natural and powerful alteration in our emotions and metabolism. Spring, for instance, stimulates us to outdoor activities, such as gardening and long walks, during which we inhale a large quantity of oxygen which helps us get rid of winter fats. Eating light foods in spring is essential to aid the liver function properly. If we ignore these signs, stay mostly indoors and maintain a winter diet, we may suffer as a consequence from mood swings, irritability and anger. The Chinese Five Element theory will show us exactly what we need to do to strengthen the flow of life in those key organs that control our well-being in each season. The accuracy of this ancient method is still a source of wonder to modern nutritionists today. Here we give readers a working, practical knowledge of the system in conjunction with the recipe section that follows. This is to maintain harmony and is not constructed to be a healing method for illness. If you are interested in finding out the medicinal properties of this system or wish to be cured from sickness, we suggest you consult a Chinese nutritionist.

Harmony with the seasons should be second nature to a balanced person; as summer draws to a close, for example, we are already aware that autumn and winter are just around the corner and so our bodies and minds make gradual arrangements, day by day. We wear warmer clothes, adjust to progressively lesser light, we begin to think about indoor activities and adopt a more contemplative mood. Each season has its beauty and magic; adjusting

THE FIVE ELEMENT CHART

SEASON	ORGANS	ELEMENT	RE-ENERGISING FOOD	FOOD CAUSING STRESS
Spring	Liver and gall bladder	Wood	SOUR TASTE Quinoa, barley, lemon, plums, daikon radishes, broccoli, cabbage, celery, carrot, parsley, sea vegetables	Alcohol, dairy products, meat, eggs, food with chemical additives
Midsummer	Heart and small intestines	Fire	BITTER TASTE Chicory, corn, spring onions, all summer vegetables, local fruit	As above
Late summer	Spleen and stomach	Earth	SWEET TASTE Pumpkin, parsnips, carrots, sweet vegetables, onions, millet, miso, kombu sea vegetable	All processed food, monosodium glutamate, fats, fruit juices
Autumn	Lungs and large intestine	Metal	SPICY TASTE Leeks, garlic, root ginger, root vegetables, brown rice, hijiki sea vegetable, miso, pears, apples	White flour, yeast, fats, antibiotics
Winter	Kidney and bladder	Water	SALTY TASTE Beans, buckwheat, sturdy green vegetables, miso, shoyu sauce, aduki beans, berries	Chilled food, raw food, sugar

to the changes around us makes us feel more in tune with nature and the bounty that is brought to us every day.

The recipes in the following section of this book are organised according to the five seasons – spring, midsummer, summer, autumn and winter. They have been carefully worked out by relating to the season's availability of fresh produce and many guidelines are given as to what cooking methods are best to employ in each season. Below is a basic chart to show the correspondences between the seasons, the elements and the organs of the body according to the Five Element theory.

Understanding the inter-connection between all the elements of the universe that surrounds us enhances our own sense of harmony and unity; we are able to flow *with* the change rather than reacting *against* it. Diet, being that part of the environment with which we directly nourish ourselves, plays a very important part in maintaining this subtle balance. Harmony means good health.

FIVE ELEMENT CORRESPONDENCES

	Five Elements	**Wood**	**Fire**	**Earth**	**Metal**	**Water**
HUMAN BODY	*Yin* Solid organ	Liver	Heart-mind	Spleen/ pancreas	Lungs	Kidneys
	Yang Hollow organ	Gallbladder	Small intestine	Stomach	Large intestine	Urinary bladder
	Sense organ Sense	Eyes/ sight	Tongues/ speech	Mouth/ taste	Nose/ smell	Ears/ hearing
	Tissue	Tendons and sinews	Blood vessels	Muscles and flesh	Skin and hair	Bones
	Emotion	Anger and impatience	Joy	Worry and anxiety	Grief and melancholy	Fear and fright
	Voice sound	Shouting	Laughing	Singing	Weeping	Groaning
	Fluid emitted	Tears	Sweat	Saliva	Mucus	Urine
		Patience	Wisdom and concentration	Giving	Vigour	Keeping moral precepts
NATURE	**Season**	**Spring**	**Midsummer**	**Late Summer**	**Autumn**	**Winter**
	Environmental influence	Wind	Heat	Dampness	Dryness	Cold
	Development	Birth	Growth	Transformation	Harvest	Storing
	Colour	Green	Red	Yellow	White	Black/dark
	Taste	Sour	Bitter	Sweet	Pungent	Salty
	Orientation	East	South	Middle	West	North
	Grain	Wheat, oats	Corn, amaranth	Millet, barley	Rice	Beans

MAKING THE TRANSITION FROM A MEAT-EATING TO A VEGETARIAN DIET

A successful transition to a vegetarian diet needs to be a gradual process; it may take months or perhaps even years until the body fully adapts to a radical switch of eating habits. If you have been eating meat all your life but would now like to switch to a vegetarian diet, we suggest you seek the help of an expert nutritionist who will discuss your individual needs and biological rhythms, so that your health is maintained throughout the transition period. Below are a few suggestions and tips. Do not rush; allow the body to make the transition at its own pace. We suggest you also read the Nutritional Supplements section listed in Chapter 10; there are many items which will help you increase the amount of plant-derived protein as you decrease protein derived from animals and dairy food.

- Gradually substitute refined grains for wholegrains – brown rice, wholewheat pasta, unrefined organically grown cereals.
- Gradually substitute products that cause loss of minerals and nutrients, such as sugar and alcohol, with natural sweeteners – honey, molasses – and more natural beverages.
- Begin using sea vegetables in your diet as they contain the whole spectrum of minerals.
- Use more vegetables and try to avoid eating red meat. Start planning your meals around the grain, pulse, vegetable axis. Progressively reduce all meat, then fish and fowl. At the same time reduce your intake of dairy food – eggs and milk.
- Sometimes combining complex carbohydrates, such as brown rice, with dairy food, causes blockages in the digestion. Keep your meals nutritious, balanced and light.
- You may find that your eating habits change quite dramatically. You may prefer to have small quantities of food often – a bowl of rice, a cup of miso soup – rather than having two gigantic meals a day. Pay attention to the energy flow in your body and mind throughout the day and perhaps draw up a chart. If you feel more hungry in the morning, then have a nutritious breakfast and a substantial lunch and end the day with a snack for dinner. Discuss these changes with your family and encourage them to chart their natural energy rhythms in a twenty-four hour cycle. Experiment and be playful, eventually you will find the perfect balance for you.

A BALANCED DIET

Attain the climax of emptiness,
preserve the utmost quiet:
as myriad things act in concert,
I thereby observe the return.
Things flourish,
then each returns to its root.
Return to the root is called stillness:
stillness is called return to Life,
return to Life is called the constant,
knowing the constant is called enlightenment.
  – Lao Tzu, from *Tao Te Ching*

The best possible diet is a balanced one. As you progressively switch from a meat-eating to a vegetarian diet you may want to plan your meals according to the proportions in the chart below. As a general rule, grains should form half of your meal, one third should be seasonal vegetables, and the last third a combination of the remaining nutrients. Also refer to the *yin–yang* chart if you want to plan your meals according to the mood or energy of the moment. Remember, grains, vegetables and pulses represent the perfectly balanced meal for any situation.

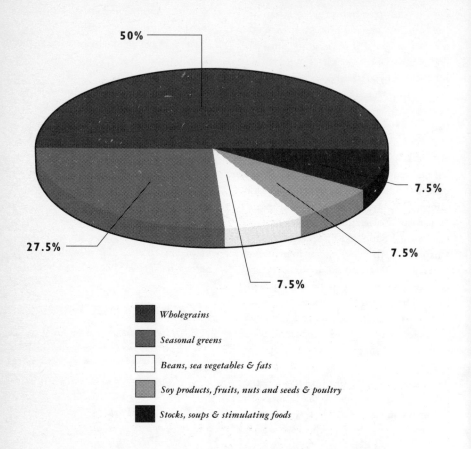

- Wholegrains
- Seasonal greens
- Beans, sea vegetables & fats
- Soy products, fruits, nuts and seeds & poultry
- Stocks, soups & stimulating foods

SUMMARY OF BASIC NUTRIENTS AND THEIR AVAILABILITY IN NATURAL SOURCES

PROTEINS	Constitute 20% of total body weight. Proteins are building blocks for muscles, blood, skin, bones, the brain and heart. They play a vital part in growth and regeneration.	Soy beans, watercress, sea vegetables, green peas, bean sprouts, broccoli, Brussel sprouts, cauliflower, kale, mushrooms, mustard.

CARBOHYDRATES	They are a source of energy and thus must constantly be supplied and replenished. Complex, slow-burning carbohydrates are the only source of fuel for the metabolism. In case of deficiency, the body breaks down proteins in order to get fuel supply.	Brown rice, barley, buckwheat, rye, bulgar wheat, oatmeal, beans, seasonal vegetables.
VITAMINS	These are micro-nutrients which need to be supplied in the diet as they are not part of the body structure. They help regulate chemical reactions within the metabolism. Vitamins that we derive from the diet can be destroyed by smoking, stress, alcohol and an excessive intake of protein. Nutritional needs of vitamins vary tremendously and change dramatically during crisis, illness, pregnancy and breast-feeding. If taken in supplements these need to be derived from a *food source* as synthetic vitamins cause toxicity in the body.	Alfalfa, apricots, carrots, oranges, winter squash, leafy greens, nuts, beans, soy food, kelp, mushrooms, bean sprouts, seeds, seasonal vegetables.
MINERALS	They play a vital role in the absorption of vitamins, regulate the pH balance of the blood and maintain the immune system. Minerals are present in the soil and are preserved in organic food.	Organic or nitrate-free of the following: raw seeds, nuts, alfalfa, pollen, brewer's yeast, kelp, molasses, black pepper, cloves, thyme.

FATS	Despite their bad reputation they are needed by the body in moderation. They help the absorption of certain vitamins and minerals. They are essential to cell structure and maintain supple skin and make hair shine.	Oils extracted from whole foods without refining. Polyunsaturated, unrefined, cold-pressed olive, corn and sesame oils are the best.
CALCIUM	This is the mineral found in bones and teeth. It regulates the heart-beat and skin balance. It is responsible for good skin and has a soothing effect on the nerves.	Sesame seeds and paste (tahini), soy beans, peanuts, green vegetables, almonds, sunflower seeds, milk, cheese.

THE IMPORTANCE OF RAW FOOD AND VEGETABLE JUICES

Raw food and fresh vegetable juices must be included in everyone's diet and should be made into a staple of everyday eating habits. They contain a broad array of vitamins, minerals and enzymes that enhance and complement individual nutrients. As raw food is not processed, they are assimilated by the body with little effort on the digestive system and have one of the strongest impacts on building our health. By adding raw food and fresh vegetable juices to a balanced diet you will improve and accelerate the process of restoring nutrients to chemically starved tissues. Spring, midsummer and summer are the obvious seasons for eating a variety of raw food; we suggest you try to include raw food, salads or carrots and celery cut into strips for dipping into sauces in all seasons. Fresh juices, made from either vegetables or fruit or a combination of the two, are vitamin bombs; they are absorbed directly into the bloodstream and are easily digested. The minerals in fresh juices are very different from those we take in supplement form because they are naturally chelated (bonded with) vitamins and amino acids and thus easily absorbed into the bloodstream. Easy-to-assimilate minerals are essential in the diet as they keep the body's energy high, the nerves calm, the muscles, heart, hair, teeth and bones strong. Try installing a juicer in your home and office and switch from compulsive coffee-drinking to juicing – you will notice an enormous difference after the first glass. Minerals help us keep the blood cleansed and its pH balanced. Juices literally transfer the vital qualities of plants and fruits directly into our bodies and they represent the most natural form, apart from water, of purified fluids which are essential to our health.

Drinking fresh juices does not tax our elimination organs – the kidneys and the liver – because the body absorbs all the nutrients directly and does not have to process harmful substances.

In the following recipe section we give recipes and suggestions for both vegetable and fruit juices that have worked again and again for us. Experiment, try your own cocktails and combinations – variety is extremely important in maintaining a healthy and balanced diet. Choose vegetables and fruit that are in season; organically grown produce is obviously the best and many suppliers sell boxes of washed-carrots and other bulk products at a slightly discounted price. Check your local suppliers and discuss your juicing programme – they will be able to make suggestions as to prices and availability of produce. If you are buying in supermarkets, choose items which have been grown locally; because you are eating them raw, you want to minimise the amount of pesticides and chemical fertilisers that have been sprayed onto your product.

RIGHT

Food, Right

EATING

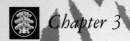

Chapter 3

RÉSUMÉ OF

RECIPES

SALAD DRESSINGS AND TOPPINGS

STOCKS

BASIC PASTRY RECIPES

BREAKFAST SUGGESTIONS

DESSERT SUGGESTIONS

FRUIT JUICE COCKTAILS

NON-DAIRY FRUIT SMOOTHIES

CHAPTER 4: SPRING

	NOTICE
	All recipes for lunch and dinner are for between 4 and 6 servings

LUNCH

DINNER

STARTERS

MAIN MEALS

CHAPTER 5: MIDSUMMER

NOTICE
All recipes for lunch and dinner are for
between 4 and 6 servings

LUNCH

DINNER

STARTERS

MAIN MEALS

CHAPTER 6: LATE SUMMER

> NOTICE
> *All recipes for lunch and dinner are for*
> *between 4 and 6 servings*

LUNCH

DINNER

STARTERS

MAIN MEALS

CHAPTER 7: AUTUMN

> NOTICE
> *All recipes for lunch and dinner are for
> between 4 and 6 servings*

LUNCH

DINNER

STARTERS

MAIN MEALS

CHAPTER 8: WINTER

LUNCH

DINNER

STARTERS

MAIN MEALS

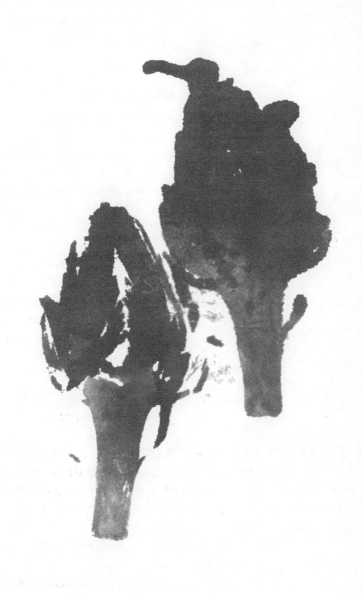

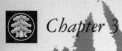

Chapter 3

THE BASICS

FLAVOURED MILKS

THESE *are two standard recipes for delicious flavoured milks. You can use any other variety of nuts — cashew, sesame seeds, walnuts, and many others — and follow the same proportions and procedure. Nuts can also be combined with fruit for a sweeter flavour; try figs, carobs, bananas or apricots. Add cinnamon, honey or maple syrup, not sugar, as sweeteners. Flavoured milks make great spring and summer thirst-quenchers and they are nutritious too. Keep them in the refrigerator and use them as alternative to cow's milk or the packaged soy milks that you find in health food stores.*

— ALMOND MILK —

100 g toasted almonds
1–2 tbsp maple syrup or honey
¼ tsp almond extract
600 ml water

SERVES 2

GRIND the almonds into a fine paste in a blender. Add sweeteners, almond extract and water and blend again for 3 or 4 minutes. Using a fine sieve or a cheesecloth, strain the almond milk slowly into a jug. Use a spoon to gently press the paste and squeeze out the milk. You will have about 2 cups of almond milk which will keep for up to 4 days in the refrigerator.

— HAZELNUT AND DATE MILK —

BLEND half the water and the other ingredients at high speed in a blender until creamy. Add remaining water and blend briefly. If you want a more liquid consistency, add 600 ml extra water – this will yield 5 cups of flavoured milk. Strain through a sieve or cheesecloth into a jug. Serve chilled. It will keep in the refrigerator for up to 4 days.

600 ml water

175 g toasted hazelnuts

100 g pitted dates

2 tsp vanilla extract

1 tbsp maple syrup

SERVES 2

SAUCES

WE *include here a large variety of sauces which can be prepared ahead of time and kept in glass or plastic containers in the refrigerator. Home-made sauces taste delicious, do not have flavourings, colourings, or preservatives and are thus a great deal more healthy than the supermarket equivalents. Take some to the office and use them as spreads on rice cakes to combat sugar cravings or to help you in low-energy periods.*

— SOUR CREAM —

STEAM the tofu for 2 minutes and then blend all the remaining ingredients, except the chives, together in a blender at high speed for 2 minutes. Remove from blender, adjust the seasoning and if necessary add more sea salt and sprinkle with the fresh chives.

140–175 g silken tofu

2 tbsp lemon juice

1 tbsp tahini

3 tsp cider vinegar

1 pinch sea salt

1 tbsp soy oil

2 tbsp fresh chives, finely chopped

MAKES 250 ml

− SUNFLOWER SOUR CREAM −

300 ml water

225 g sunflower seeds

1 tsp sea salt

4 tbsp lemon juice

½ tsp each onion and garlic powder

MAKES 250 ml

BLEND all the ingredients together in a blender at high speed for 2–3 minutes. Remove from blender and adjust for salt. Keeps in the refrigerator for up to 4 days.

− TOFU MAYONNAISE −

225 g crumbled firm tofu

4 tbsp water

½ tsp sea salt

1 tsp lemon juice

1 tsp brewer's yeast (optional)

½ tsp each onion and garlic powder

4 tbsp rape seed oil

½ tsp cider vinegar

MAKES 250 ml

BLEND all the ingredients together in a blender at high speed for 3–4 minutes until creamy. Remove from blender and adjust for salt. Keeps in the refrigerator for up to 4 days.

− ALMOND MAYONNAISE −

250 g toasted almonds

170 ml soy milk

¼ tsp garlic powder

1 pinch sea salt

300 ml safflower oil

3 tbsp lemon juice

½ tsp cider vinegar

MAKES 250 ml

REMOVE the skin from the toasted almonds and grind them to a fine paste. Add all the other ingredients except the last three to the blender and blend until smooth and creamy. With the blender still running, add the oil, pouring it in a slow, steady stream; next add the lemon juice, then the vinegar in the same fashion.

If the sauce has not thickened to your liking after you have poured the oil into the blender, pour into a pan and cook on a medium heat, stirring constantly, until thickened. In this case add the lemon juice and the vinegar only after you have removed the pan from the heat. Add seasoning and herbs of your choice. Keeps up to 10 days in the refrigerator.

— SOY GARLIC MAYONNAISE —

BLEND first three ingredients. With blender still running, add oil in a slow, steady stream. Add lemon juice and blend for a further 2 minutes. Remove from blender and refrigerate.

300 ml soy milk
½ tsp sea salt
2 garlic cloves, crushed
300 ml safflower oil
2 tbsp lemon juice

MAKES 600 ml

— TOFU RUSSIAN DRESSING —

PLACE tofu in a blender and blend until smooth. Then combine with the rest of the ingredients and blend until smooth and creamy. Keep refrigerated.

225 g firm tofu
4 tbsp tomato ketchup
1 tbsp tahini
4 tbsp lemon juice
1 tsp dried dill
4 tbsp grated carrot and parsley

MAKES 300 ml

— TOFU COTTAGE CHEESE —

BLEND half of the tofu with the rest of the ingredients until smooth. Remove from blender and place in a bowl. Mash the other half of the tofu in a separate bowl with a fork until crumbly and add to the blended mix. Test for salt and refrigerate.

450 g firm tofu
1 tbsp cider vinegar
2 tbsp lemon juice
225 g finely chopped onions
2 tsp chopped fresh parsley
1 pinch sea salt

MAKES 450 g

BASIC SPREADS AND DIPS

DIPS *are an easy and healthy hors-d'oeuvre for cock-tail parties or everyday snacks. Cut up celery, carrot and cucumber sticks to dip. Spreads are great on rice or oat-meal cakes. Make your own and keep in the refrigerator at home or in the office.*

— HOUMMUS —

1 tbsp olive oil
225 g finely chopped onion
(optional)
4 garlic cloves, crushed
450 g cooked chickpeas (can also used tinned)
juice of 2 lemons
150 ml tahini
¼ tsp cayenne pepper
4 tbsp water from cooking the chickpeas (or ordinary water if using tinned)

MAKES 450 g

HEAT the oil and sauté the onion and garlic until tender. Blend the rest of the ingredients in a blender at high speed until smooth and creamy. If using it just as a dressing for salads or grains, increase the amount of water. Blend the sautéed onion and garlic with the rest of the mix. Keep refrigerated.

— GUACAMOLE —

Mix all the ingredients well. Check seasoning and serve immediately or keep refrigerated for up to 2 days.

For quick guacamole, you can use ½ tsp each garlic and onion powder and 2 tbsp of tomato purée instead of fresh garlic, onion and tomato.

450 g ripe and mashed avocado

2 garlic cloves, crushed

½ onion, finely chopped

225 g tomatoes, finely chopped

1 tbsp lemon juice

½ tsp ground cumin

½ tsp each cayenne pepper and sea salt

100 g fresh chopped coriander

4 tbsp fresh parsley, chopped

MAKES 450 g

— SALSA —

Combine all the ingredients together. Keep refrigerated for up to 2 days. This is a great dip for corn and blue corn tortilla chips.

4 plum tomatoes, diced, or 800 g canned whole tomatoes

175 g finely chopped green pepper (1 pepper)

1 tbsp finely crushed garlic

100 g red onion, finely chopped

2 tsp cider vinegar

2 tsp ground cumin

2 tbsp minced coriander

1 fresh chilli pepper, finely chopped

1 pinch each sea salt and pepper

honey (if chilli is unbearably hot for you)

MAKES 600 ml

– BABA GHANOUJ –

1 aubergine
4 tbsp lemon juice
4 tbsp tahini
2 garlic cloves, finely crushed
1 tbsp olive oil
4 tbsp fresh parsley, finely chopped
1 pinch each sea salt and pepper
2 spring onions, finely chopped

MAKES 450 g

PRE-HEAT the oven to 200°C/400°F/Gas Mark 6. Using a fork, prick the aubergine all over, place it in a baking dish and transfer to the hot oven. Bake for about 45 minutes or until crinkly on the outside and soft on the inside. Allow the aubergine to cool until you can handle it safely. Remove the skin and scoop out the inside.

Chop or purée the aubergine with the other ingredients except for the parsley and spring onions which you can add to the dish when cool and ready to serve. The aubergine can also be char-grilled on a skewer over an open flame – this gives it a distinct and delicious smoky taste. Keep refrigerated.

– ARTICHOKE SPREAD –

6–8 artichokes
2 tbsp olive oil
1 tbsp wine vinegar
2 garlic cloves, crushed
1 tbsp lemon juice
1 pinch each sea salt and pepper

MAKES 450 g

REMOVE the stalks and the tough outer leaves from the artichokes. Place them in a large pan with water and boil gently for 45 minutes. Remove them from the water and allow them to cool.

Discard the remaining tough leaves and scrape the soft, edible flesh from the bottom of the leaves and place in the blender with the soft artichoke centres.

Blend the artichoke flesh with the rest of the ingredients in a blender until smooth and creamy. Season well, chill and serve on toast.

SALAD DRESSINGS

WE *give here a variety of dressings to use for salads and with any cooked grains combination — millet, quinoa, barley, brown basmati rice, or kashi. They can all be made ahead of time and refrigerated. Keep these dressings at the office too to be used over take-away salads or rice. Ready-made salad dressings from supermarkets are invariably more fattening as they contain preservatives, colourings and flavourings; they are also more expensive.*

— DAIRY-FREE THOUSAND ISLAND DRESSING —

BLEND all the ingredients well in a blender until smooth and creamy. You can also use chopped black olives and grated carrots to make a different variation of this delicious Thousand Island Dressing. Keep refrigerated.

300 ml dairy-free mayonnaise
4 tbsp tomato ketchup
1 tbsp spring onions, finely chopped
2 tsp finely chopped fresh parsley
1 tbsp grated green pepper
2 tbsp grated dill pickle
1 tsp lemon juice

MAKES 900 ml

— FRENCH DRESSING —

4 tbsp extra-virgin olive oil
1 garlic clove, finely crushed
1½ tsp Dijon mustard
2 tbsp lemon juice
150 ml vegetable juice or water
1 tbsp honey
4 tbsp fresh parsley, finely
chopped
1 pinch each sea salt and pepper

MAKES 300 ml

BLEND all the ingredients at high speed in a blender. Keep refrigerated.

— ITALIAN DRESSING —

4 tbsp extra-virgin olive oil
1 tbsp lemon juice
150 ml water or tomato juice
1 garlic clove, crushed
1 tbsp finely chopped onion
1 tbsp fresh basil, in fine strips
1 tsp oregano
1 tbsp tomato purée
1 tbsp balsamic vinegar

MAKES 300 ml

MIX all the ingredients well. Keep refrigerated.

— GARLIC AND TAHINI DRESSING —

BLEND all the ingredients together except for the herbs which can be added just before serving. Keep refrigerated.

1½ tbsp extra-virgin olive oil
1 garlic clove, finely crushed
2 tbsp lemon or lime juice
4 tbsp tahini
6 tbsp water
1 tbsp soy sauce
1 tbsp cider vinegar
4 tbsp water
1 pinch black pepper
fresh mixed herbs, to flavour

MAKES 150 ml

— CARROT AND GINGER DRESSING —

BLEND all the ingredients well in a blender. Keep refrigerated.

150 ml carrot juice
½ tsp root ginger, finely chopped
2 tsp lemon juice
3 tbsp tahini
½ tsp curry powder
2 tbsp fresh coriander, chopped
½ to 1 tsp of honey or maple syrup
2 tbsp sesame oil (optional)
1 pinch each sea salt and pepper

MAKES 175 ml

– GREEN DRESSING –

1 plum tomato, finely chopped
100 g fresh arugula or spinach,
finely chopped
2 tbsp lemon juice
4 tbsp water or vegetable juice
2 garlic cloves, crushed
2 tbsp soy sauce
1 tsp chopped fresh oregano
2 tsp honey
4 tbsp extra-virgin olive oil
1 pinch each sea salt and pepper

MAKES 300 ml

PLACE all the ingredients in a blender and blend until smooth and creamy. If the dressing is too thick for your liking, strain it through a fine sieve. Keep refrigerated.

– SWEET AND GINGERY DRESSING –

6 shallots, peeled and finely
chopped
1 tbsp root ginger, finely chopped
4 tbsp fresh mint, finely chopped
4 tbsp pineapple juice
4 tbsp water
1 tsp rice vinegar
2 tbsp walnut oil
1 pinch each sea salt and pepper

MAKES 300 ml

HEAT the oil and sauté the shallots for 5 or 6 minutes. Transfer to the blender and blend all the ingredients at high speed. Keep refrigerated.

— SUNFLOWER SEED DRESSING —

COMBINE the char-grilled tomatoes with the sun-dried tomatoes in a blender and blend. Add the remaining ingredients and blend until finely minced but not smooth. Keep refrigerated.

2 large tomatoes, grilled, charred and skinned
4 tbsp sun-dried tomatoes
4 tbsp sunflower seeds, toasted
4 tbsp orange juice
4 tbsp water
¼ tsp honey
¼ tsp mustard
¼ tsp soy sauce
1 pinch black pepper

MAKES 300 ml

— CREAMY MUSTARD DRESSING —

MIX all the ingredients in a blender until smooth and creamy. You can adjust the consistency with a little more water according to what use you are going to make of the dressing. Keep refrigerated.

100 g firm tofu
6 tbsp extra-virgin olive oil
1 garlic clove, finely crushed
2 tbsp tomato ketchup or tomato purée
2 tsp soy sauce
4 tbsp vegetable juice or water
1 tsp mustard
3 tbsp lemon juice
1 celery stick, finely chopped
1 tbsp cider vinegar
3 spring onions, finely chopped
chopped fresh chives or dill, to flavour
1 pinch each sea salt and pepper

MAKES 300 ml

— MANGO AND GINGER SALAD
DRESSING —

150 ml mango juice
4 tbsp diced mango
1 tsp freshly grated root
ginger juice
1 tsp fresh lime juice
4 tbsp water
1/4 tsp cayenne pepper
2 tbsp finely chopped spring
onions
1 tbsp fresh coriander
1 pinch sea salt

MAKES 300 ml

BLEND all the ingredients in a blender. Keep refrigerated.

— WALNUT OIL AND FRESH JUICE
DRESSING —

5 tbsp orange juice
5 tbsp grapefruit juice
4 tbsp water
1/2 tsp grated lemon rind
1 tsp champagne vinegar
3 spring onions, finely chopped
1/4 tsp dill seeds, crushed
1 tbsp walnut oil
chopped fresh herbs, to flavour
1 pinch each sea salt and pepper

MAKES 170 ml

WHISK all the ingredients together and adjust the seasoning. Keep refrigerated.

— ROASTED RED PEPPER TOPPING —

CHAR the pepper under a grill, turning it so that all sides are evenly grilled. Place the pepper in a covered container — the moisture released from its heat will make the skin easier to remove. Peel the skin off, remove the seeds and ribs.

Blend the pepper with the rest of the ingredients in a blender until smooth. Keep refrigerated.

1 large red pepper
1 garlic clove, finely crushed
1 tbsp extra-virgin olive oil
1 tsp sherry vinegar
4 tbsp water
2 tsp chopped fresh basil and oregano
10 sultanas, soaked in warm water for a few minutes
1 pinch each sea salt and pepper

MAKES 170 ml

— CREAMY ORIENTAL DRESSING —

COMBINE all the ingredients in a blender to make a creamy, nutty dressing. Keep refrigerated.

4 tbsp light sesame oil
¼ cup pine nuts
1 tbsp fresh coriander
1 tsp finely chopped root ginger
1 tsp soy sauce
1 tsp lemon juice
2 tbsp grated coconut
1–2 tbsp water

MAKES 300 ml

— CUCUMBER AND DILL DRESSING —

BLEND all the ingredients until smooth and creamy. Keep refrigerated.

2 tbsp dairy-free sour cream
4 tbsp water
100 g chopped fresh dill
1 cucumber, peeled and segmented in 10 cm slices
2 garlic cloves, crushed
¼ tsp mustard powder
1 tbsp finely chopped red onion
1 pinch each sea salt and pepper

MAKES 300 ml

— TOMATO DRESSING —

150 ml tomato juice
4 tbsp water
1 garlic clove, finely crushed
1 tbsp chopped fresh basil
1 tbsp mustard
½ tsp honey
1 pinch each sea salt and pepper

MAKES 300 ml

BLEND all the ingredients together. Keep refrigerated.

—LEMON VINAIGRETTE —

6 tbsp extra-virgin olive oil
3 tbsp lemon juice
4 tbsp water
2 tbsp sour cream or mayonnaise
½ tsp chopped fresh tarragon
1 tbsp sherry vinegar
1 tsp mustard
1 pinch each sea salt and pepper

MAKES 170 ml

BLEND all the ingredients together. Keep refrigerated.

— CAPER AND BLACK OLIVE DRESSING —

1 red pepper, roasted and puréed
4 tbsp water
1 garlic clove, finely crushed
1 tsp onion powder
100 g pitted black olives, sliced
1 tbsp chopped small capers
3 spring onions, finely chopped
1 tbsp finely chopped fresh parsley
1 tbsp Balsamic vinegar

MAKES 170 ml

COMBINE and blend all the ingredients in a bowl. Keep refrigerated.

BEETROOT AND HORSERADISH DRESSING

BLEND the first five ingredients in a blender. Add the sesame seeds, fresh herbs and seasoning at the last minute. Keep refrigerated.

4 tbsp extra-virgin olive oil
1 beetroot, cooked and shredded
1 tsp chopped fresh horseradish
1 tbsp wine vinegar
4 tbsp water
1 tbsp white sesame seeds, toasted
chopped fresh herbs, to flavour
1 pinch each sea salt and pepper

MAKES 170 ml

—PEANUT AND COCONUT SAUCE —

WHISK and blend all the ingredients together until smooth. Keep refrigerated.

1 tbsp crunchy peanut butter
1 tsp root ginger, finely chopped
4 tbsp coconut cream
2 tbsp stock
2 tsp soy sauce
4 tbsp water
2 tsp finely chopped spring onions

MAKES 170 ml

— CREAMY SPINACH DRESSING —

BLEND all the ingredients and adjust for seasoning. Keep refrigerated.

8 spinach leaves, chopped
2 tbsp finely chopped fresh parsley
1 tsp honey
2 tbsp lemon juice
1 tbsp roughly chopped walnuts
6 tbsp extra-virgin olive oil or walnut oil
1 garlic clove, finely crushed
8 tbsp soy cream (non-dairy cream)

MAKES 170 ml

— PESTO AND CARROT DRESSING —

4 tbsp ready-made pesto
150 ml fresh carrot juice
4 tbsp soy milk, plain flavour
4 tbsp roughly chopped walnuts
½ tsp soy sauce
2 tbsp extra-virgin olive oil
(optional)
1 pinch pepper

MAKES 300 ml

WHISK all the ingredients together for a quick and delicious salad dressing. Keep refrigerated.

— JAPANESE PLUM DRESSING —

2 tbsp sesame oil
1 tsp umeboshi plum paste
(umeboshi are Japanese pickled
salted plums, available from
health food stores)
1 tbsp mirin (sweet rice vinegar)
4 tbsp water
1 tbsp soy sauce
½ tsp finely chopped root ginger
1 small tomato, finely chopped
2 spring onions, finely chopped
chopped fresh parsley, to flavour

MAKES 170 ml

WHISK all the ingredients together. Sprinkle with black sesame seeds and nori flakes if you wish. Keep refrigerated.

— MISO AND GINGER DRESSING —

COMBINE all the ingredients well using a whisk. Keep refrigerated.

2 tbsp red miso paste

1 tbsp mirin (sweet rice vinegar)

½ tsp chopped root ginger

1 tbsp gomasio (a condiment made from roasted sesame seeds and sea salt, available from health food stores)

2 tbsp tahini

1½ tsp soy sauce

1–2 tbsp water

MAKES 170 ml

— PUMPKIN SEED DRESSING —

BLEND all the ingredients in a blender until smooth and creamy. Add more water if you want a thinner consistency. Keep refrigerated.

225 g finely chopped fresh parsley

4 tbsp pumpkin seeds

¼–½ cup water

2 tbsp lemon juice

1 garlic clove, finely chopped

1 tbsp sunflower oil

1 pinch each sea salt and pepper

MAKES 170 ml

— CURRY DRESSING —

WHISK all the ingredients well. Keep refrigerated.

2 garlic cloves, crushed

1 tsp finely chopped root ginger

½ tsp each ground cumin and coriander

1 tbsp lemon juice

4 tbsp extra-virgin olive oil

½ tsp curry powder

2 tbsp tahini

4 tbsp water

1 pinch each sea salt and pepper

MAKES 170 ml

STOCKS

HERE *are two recipes for good everyday stocks. You can change the vegetables in the recipe for the basic stock according to the seasons, e.g. pumpkin in autumn, or seasonal greens.*

— BASIC STOCK —

2 onions, quartered
2 carrots, cut in 2.5 cm pieces
2 leeks, chopped
1 potato, cubed
2 garlic cloves, chopped
handful of greens
only if available in season or
mushroom stems
1 bay leaf
4 peppercorns
2 cloves
1 bunch fresh parsley
½ tsp each chopped fresh
marjoram and thyme
1 litre water
1 tsp sea salt

MAKES 1 litre

ROUGHLY clean and chop all the vegetables, leaving the skin on wherever possible. Combine all the ingredients in a large pot, cover with the water, bring it to the boil and simmer covered for 45 minutes to 1½ hours, stirring occasionally.

Remove from heat when cooked, allow it to cool to room temperature and strain through a sieve. For a more potent stock, simmer the broth until it is reduced to half its original quantity. This stock can be refrigerated for up to 5 days.

Variations and suggestions:

- For a richer stock, sauté vegetables in 2 tbsp extra-virgin olive oil at the start.
- For tomato soup, reduce water and add 450 g–1 kg fresh chopped tomatoes with some rice syrup.
- To sweeten the stock, add slices of apples and pears.
- For mushroom soup, add 450 g fresh shiitake and button mushrooms with 150 ml white wine.
- For a Mediterranean Stock add fresh basil, more parsley, pesto, more garlic and white wine.
- For a Curry Stock add a tsp each of ground coriander, cumin and turmeric.

— JAPANESE STOCK —

SOAK the kombu and shiitake mushrooms in warm water for 2–3 hours. Bring the water to the boil, lower the heat and add all the other ingredients, simmering for 15–20 minutes. Keep refrigerated for up to 5 days.

Variation:

For Thai Stock: add grated root ginger, lemon grass, sweet basil and chillies.

20 cm piece kombu, cut into strips
4 dried shiitake mushrooms
1 litre water
2 tbsp sea salt
3 tbsp soy sauce
2 tbsp sugar
2 tbsp mirin (sweet rice vinegar)
2 tsp sake
4 spring onions, finely chopped
1 tsp wasabi paste
1 carrot, finely chopped

MAKES 1 litre

BASIC PASTRY RECIPES

— PASTRY DOUGH OR PIE CRUST —

SIFT the flour and salt. Add cold margarine with a pastry knife or grate it. Work it into the flour until the mixture resembles breadcrumbs. Add cold water gradually, a tablespoon at a time, mixing all the while until the dough forms into a ball. Be careful not to over-handle it. Use your hands or a fork to mix.

Wrap the dough in waxed paper, place it inside a sealed plastic food bag and refrigerate for up to a week.

Roll out the dough into a medium pie dish. For best results, freeze the shaped dough inside the pie dish for at least 1 hour before baking it.

If baking without a filling, preheat the oven to 200°C/400°F/Gas Mark 6, and transfer the frozen pie crust to the hot oven for 15–20 minutes. The crust can be lined with foil to keep it from cracking and the centre filled with dried beans to weigh it down and prevent it from becoming soggy. Bake it until lightly browned.

250 g wholewheat pastry flour
1 pinch sea salt
6 tbsp soy margarine
4–5 tbsp iced water

1¼ *tbsp dried yeast*
4-6 *tbsp warm water*
1 *pinch sugar*
225 g *wholewheat flour*
275 g *unbleached white flour*
½ *tsp sea salt*
3 *tbsp extra-virgin olive oil*

COMBINE the yeast, warm water and sugar, stir to dissolve and activate the yeast.

Mix together the two types of flour on a large, clean working surface and make a small well in the centre. Pour in the yeast mix, the salt and a tablespoon of oil. Start sifting flour into the well carefully with your hands, kneading all the time until the dough becomes a ball. Continue kneading for a further 8–10 minutes until the dough is moist and elastic. Add more water if needed as you work with the dough.

Put the dough in an oiled bowl, turning it over once so that the whole surface is oiled on all sides. Cover the dough with a clean towel and keep it in a warm place (preferably in the sun) to rise to double its size, approximately 60–80 minutes.

Preheat the oven to 200°C/400°F/Gas Mark 6.

If using a pizza pan, oil it well. Roll out the pizza dough on a floured surface to half of its final size. Place the dough in the pan and slowly stretch it to the sides and over the borders. Best size is 25 cm round and about 3 cm thick. Top it with your favourite ingredients and bake for 30 minutes.

BREAKFAST SUGGESTIONS

— APPLE AND CINNAMON MUFFINS —

PREHEAT the oven to 190°C/375°F/Gas Mark 5. Grease a muffin tray. Mix oil, honey and apple sauce well. Sift together the rest of the dry ingredients, including the raisins. Stir wet ingredients into dry. Don't over-mix, the mixture should be lumpy. Drop into muffin holes and bake for 20 minutes. Cool muffins on a wire rack.

When you put the muffin tray into the oven, put in an oven-proof bowl with water as it helps to keep the muffins moist.

4 tbsp sunflower oil

4 tbsp honey

300 ml apple sauce

275 g wholewheat flour

½ tsp baking soda

1½ tsp baking powder

¾ tsp allspice

¼ tsp cinnamon

½ tsp salt

100 g raisins

MAKES 12 MUFFINS

— BANANA AND BRAN MUFFINS —

PREHEAT the oven 190°C/375°F/Gas Mark 5. Blend together tofu, egg, bananas, oil and maple syrup. In another bowl, sift all the dry ingredients. Make a well in the middle of the bowl, pour in banana mix and fold in with a spatula until everything is thoroughly mixed. Spoon the batter into an oiled muffin tray and bake for 25 minutes. Cool on a wire rack.

2 tbsp mashed tofu

2 egg whites, or 1 egg

275 g mashed ripe bananas

4 tbsp sunflower oil

5 tbsp maple syrup

pinch of salt

225 g wholewheat flour

175 g oat bran

2 tsp baking powder

½ tsp baking soda

1 pinch cinnamon

1 pinch nutmeg or a few cloves

MAKES 12 TO 14 MUFFINS

– WALNUT AND DATE MUFFINS –

450 g wholewheat flour
175 g unbleached white flour
1 tbsp baking powder
1 pinch sea salt
4 egg whites
300 ml soy milk
150 ml sunflower oil
150 ml honey
225 g chopped dates
100 g chopped walnuts

MAKES 12 MUFFINS

PREHEAT oven to 190°C/375°F/Gas Mark 5. Sift all the dry ingredients together. Mix together all wet ingredients with a whisk. Mix dates and nuts into dry ingredients and then fold them into wet ingredients. Work all the ingredients well until they are thoroughly mixed. Spoon the mixture into an oiled muffin tray and bake for 25 minutes. Cool on a wire rack.

– CRACKED WHEAT PORRIDGE –

225 g cracked wheat
900 ml vanilla-flavoured soy milk
600 ml water
100 g sultanas
4 tbsp chopped apricots
3 tbsp honey
4 tbsp toasted almonds

MAKES 675 g

IN a medium-sized pan dry-roast the cracked wheat until its flavour comes out. Keep stirring the wheat until slightly brown. Add 600 ml of milk and 600 ml of water together with the sultanas, mix well and bring to the boil. Lower heat and simmer, stirring frequently, for 15 minutes or until all the moisture is absorbed. Turn off the heat and leave the pot covered to rest for 10 minutes. Warm remaining milk and honey and pour over the porridge together with the toasted almonds. Serve warm in individual bowls.

– FIG AND OAT PORRIDGE –

450 g raw oat groats, soaked 48 hours and rinsed every day
5 figs, soaked overnight
coconut, for sprinkling

MAKES 900 g

AFTER 48 hours, rinse and drain the oat groats. Put them in a blender together with the figs. Blend until smooth. Pour this mixture onto a baking tray, sprinkle with coconut and bake in a preheated oven for 1 hour at 180°C/350°F/Gas Mark 4.

— BROWN RICE PORRIDGE —

Mix all ingredients and pour onto an oiled baking dish. Bake in a preheated oven for 45 and 60 minutes at 180°C/350°F/Gas Mark 4, depending on the consistency you require. To keep it creamy, add more milk.

225 g cooked brown rice
225 g cooked barley
600 ml nut or soy milk
100 g chopped mixed nuts
100 g sultanas
4 tbsp chopped dates
½ tsp lemon juice
2 tbsp honey
1 pinch sea salt
1 pinch ground cinnamon
½ tsp vanilla essence

MAKES 900 g

— MUESLI —

Preheat the oven to 160°C/325°F/Gas Mark 3. In a bowl combine the oats, almonds, pumpkin seeds and dried coconut. Combine oil, syrup, vanilla, almond extract, spices and a little salt. Heat the mixture in a saucepan until it is watery. Pour this mix over the dry ingredients, tossing until everything is moistened. It is best mixed by your hands wearing disposable gloves. Spread the mixture on a baking tray and bake for 20 minutes, stirring every 5 minutes until the mix becomes evenly golden. Transfer to a cool tray or a bowl and toss until cool. Add the dried fruit to the cooled mix and store in an airtight container.

900 g rolled oats
175 g chopped almonds
100 g pumpkin seeds
100 g dried coconut
4 tbsp sunflower oil
150 ml maple syrup
1 tsp vanilla essence
½ tsp almond extract
1 tsp ground cinnamon
225 g mixed fruit – dried apricots, prunes, figs, papaya, or mango

MAKES 400g

– WAFFLES –

225 g wholewheat flour
100 g unbleached white flour
4 tbsp rice flour
3 tsp baking powder
¼ tsp sea salt
4 egg whites, beaten
350 ml soy milk
1 tsp vanilla extract
150 ml sunflower oil
450 g chopped fresh fruit or nuts
maple syrup, to serve
butter, to serve

MAKES 4–5 WAFFLES

PREHEAT a waffle iron and oil it with a brush. Mix together the dry ingredients. Add wet ingredients, adding the oil last. Don't over mix. Pour the mix onto a hot waffle iron and cook until waffles are golden brown, about 6–7 minutes. Serve them warm with maple syrup and fresh fruit.

– PANCAKES –

1 litre soy milk
2 tbsp honey
100 g poppy seeds
450 g wholewheat flour
1 tsp sea salt
½ tsp baking soda
4 egg whites, beaten
4 tbsp sunflower oil
1 tbsp maple flavouring
Maple syrup, to serve

MAKES 15–18 PANCAKES

HEAT 500 ml of soy milk. When it is nearly boiling, add the honey and poppy seeds, remove from the heat and set aside to cool. Mix all dry ingredients in a bowl and blend gradually with wet ingredients – the milk with honey and poppy seeds, the remaining milk and 2 tbsp of sunflower oil – except for the maple syrup. Heat a lightly oiled skillet over a medium heat. When hot, add several spoonfuls of batter, spreading it with the bottom of a round spoon. When the edges are cooked and the bottom brown, flip and cook the other side for another 2–3 minutes. Serve the pancakes warm with warmed maple syrup or any fresh fruit topping or soy cream.

— SUNDAY SUMPTUOUS BREAKFAST — BAKED EGGS WITH HASH BROWN WAFFLES AND GRILLED TOMATOES AND MUSHROOMS —

SERVE this breakfast with ketchup and mustard and wholewheat toast.

For the baked eggs:
sunflower oil
2 tbsp tomato ketchup
2 tsp prepared mustard
2 spring onions, chopped
2–3 eggs
1 pinch each sea salt and pepper
chopped fresh coriander

PREHEAT the oven to 160°C/325°F/Gas Mark 3. Butter or oil two or three cups in a muffin-tray. Mix the tomato ketchup, mustard and spring onions. Drop this mixture on the bottom of each cup of the muffin-tray and crack an egg on top. Sprinkle lightly with salt, pepper and fresh coriander. Place the tray in the oven and bake for 8–10 minutes depending on how you like your eggs. When ready, turn them out onto a hot plate with the help of a knife.

For the tomatoes and mushrooms:
2 tbsp olive oil
375 g mushrooms, quartered
1 tsp each fresh parsley, sea salt and pepper
2 tomatoes, cut into halves

HEAT the oil in a pan on a moderate heat. Add mushrooms, half the parsley, salt and pepper. Stir and sauté until lightly brown. Move them to the side of the pan and add the tomatoes. Drizzle them with a little olive oil and the rest of the parsley. Alternatively, the tomatoes can be put under a grill.

For the hash brown waffles:
2 tbsp olive oil
1 onion, finely chopped
1 tsp dried dill
800 g potatoes, shredded
handful fresh parsley, finely chopped
1 pinch each sea salt and pepper
SERVES 2

PREHEAT a waffle machine and oil liberally. In a frying pan, heat the oil and sauté the onion with the dry dill for 5 minutes. Mix in the potatoes, parsley and seasoning and place mixture in the heated and oiled waffle iron. Close the lid and let it cook for 10–12 minutes until browned.

— VEGAN HIGH PROTEIN SUNDAY BREAKFAST — SCRAMBLED TOFU WITH BAKED BEANS AND SAVOURY FLAKED PUFFED RICE —

For the scrambled tofu:
2 tbsp olive oil
175 g onion, finely chopped
1 garlic clove, chopped
¼ tsp curry powder (optional)
1 carrot, grated
1 stick celery, thinly sliced
¼ tsp each sea salt and pepper
4 tbsp diced fresh tomato
450 g firm tofu, mashed
1 tbsp chopped fresh parsley

HEAT the oil in a large frying pan and sauté onion and garlic. Add curry powder, if using. Next add carrot and celery. Sprinkle with seasonings. Continue cooking until vegetables are almost soft. Add tomato and tofu. Stir together or use a potato mash. Mix the ingredients well until dry. Serve hot with a sprinkling of fresh parsley.

PREHEAT the oven to 180°C/350°F/Gas Mark 4. Sauté onion, garlic and tofu for 2 minutes in the oil. Combine rest of the ingredients together, stir in the sautéed onion and tofu mix, add some water from the beans so as not to be too dry. Season well. Transfer the mix to an oven-proof dish, cover and bake for ½ hour. Uncover, add more bean water if dry and cook for a further 14 minutes. Sprinkle with gomasio and serve on toast.

For the baked beans:

1 diced onion

1 garlic clove, chopped

2 tbsp firm tofu, mashed

2 tbsp oil

450 g cooked navy beans – save

300 ml of the cooking liquid

4 tbsp chopped pimientos

2 tbsp tomato purée

1 tsp prepared mustard

1 pinch each sea salt and pepper

1 tsp honey

gomasio, to sprinkle (a seasoning made from ground sesame seeds and sea salt, available in health food shops)

HEAT oil in a wok over a moderate heat, add mustard seeds, reduce heat and cover until the splutter of seeds stops. Add onion together with turmeric and coriander. Fry until translucent. To the onion, add the rest of the vegetables with a hint of water. Mix well and cook for 6-8 minutes. Soak the puffed rice in cold water for 5 minutes. Drain and add to the cooking vegetables. Sprinkle over curry powder, salt and pepper. Mix well. Let it cook for a further 8 minutes. Stir and toss the mix well. When ready, transfer to a serving dish. Sprinkle with chopped peanuts, fresh coriander and lemon juice.

For the savoury flaked puffed rice:

2 tbsp vegetable oil

1 tsp mustard seeds

1 onion, sliced

¼ tsp turmeric

¼ tsp dried coriander

1 carrot, diced

100 g green peas or small cauliflower florets

225 g puffed rice (available from health food stores)

¼ tsp curry powder

4 tbsp chopped roasted peanuts

1 tbsp fresh coriander

2 tbsp lemon juice

SERVES 2

FRUIT BREAKFASTS

FRUIT *breakfasts are deliciously light and provide all the sweetness one craves in the morning. Always choose fruits that are in season and drink a fruit or vegetable juice cocktail for a vitamin-packed start to the day. All recipes below serve one.*

— FRUIT SALAD WITH MINT —

seasonal fruits, peeled and thinly sliced
300 ml live yoghurt
few mint leaves, torn

MIX the fruit with the yoghurt and sprinkle the torn mint leaves on top. The juice from the fruit will make this mixture creamy and light.

— STRAWBERRIES AND NUT CREAM —

soy cream
hazelnuts, almonds or walnuts
strawberries

BLEND the soy cream with your choice of nuts until creamy and smooth. Pour over the strawberries.

— FRESH BERRIES WITH MAPLE SYRUP —

raspberries, cloudberries, loganberries, blackberries, redcurrants, or blackcurrants
ratural maple syrup

THIS is a great late-summer breakfast dish – choose berries that are still firm as they are the sweetest. Pour over maple syrup.

— APPLE, CELERY AND NUT DELIGHT —

MIX the ingredients thoroughly.

1½ apples – Golden Delicious,
Granny Smith or organic apples
of your choice, finely sliced
1 celery stick, finely sliced
hazelnuts, almonds or walnuts,
finely chopped
300 ml live yoghurt

DESSERT SUGGESTIONS

— BROWN RICE PUDDING —

PREHEAT the oven to 180°C/350°F/Gas Mark 4. Wash and drain the rice well. Place it in a heavy pan with soy milk and the cinnamon stick and simmer gently for 1 hour. Remove the cinnamon stick and transfer the rice to an oven-proof dish, add the rest of the ingredients and bake for 25 minutes. Serve warm or at room temperature.

100 g brown rice
750 ml vanilla-flavoured soy milk
1 stick cinnamon
4 tbsp sultanas
4 tbsp chopped apricots
4 tbsp almonds, slivered

SERVES 2

— FIRNEE —

SET the vanilla-flavoured soy milk to boil over a medium heat. As the milk heats up, add the cardamom seeds and the maple syrup. Stir well and bring to the boil. Remove the milk from the heat and pour, in a thin stream, into the rice flour and milk mix. Using a whisk, work the milk and the rice paste together. Return the mix to the heat and simmer for a further 15 minutes on a low heat. Remove from the heat and pour into individual bowls. Sprinkle with chopped nuts and allow it to cool. Serve chilled or at room temperature.

600 ml vanilla-flavoured soy milk
⅛ tsp cardamom seeds, crushed
4 tbsp maple syrup
5 tsp rice flour mixed with 3 tbsp
soy milk
2 tbsp chopped mixed nuts

SERVES 2

— STRAWBERRY COUSCOUS CAKE —

225 g couscous
450 ml almond amazake
(Japanese sweetener made from
sweet rice. It can also be used as a
refreshing drink. Available from
health food stores in different
flavours.)
150 ml water
5 tbsp apple juice
1 tsp vanilla essence

For the topping:
225 g strawberries, cut into
halves (you can also use other
seasonal berries – blueberries,
raspberries, etc.)
1 tbsp kuzu (a non-flavoured
white root starch available from
health food stores and Japanese
supermarkets)
175 ml apple juice
½ tsp grated lemon zest
½ tsp vanilla extract

SERVES 4

COMBINE the couscous with the amazake, water, apple juice and vanilla in a saucepan over a medium heat. Stir for 10 minutes or until couscous starts swelling up.

Arrange this mix in an oven-proof dish. Even the surface with a spatula. Arrange strawberry halves artistically over the base. Dissolve the kuzu into the apple juice, add lemon zest and vanilla and heat on a low heat until the sauce begins to thicken. Pour this mix evenly over the cake. Cool in the refrigerator before serving.

— APPLES AND PEARS —

PUT raisins and water in a pan over a medium heat. Bring to the boil and simmer for 8–10 minutes. Add the sliced fruit, cover and simmer until the fruit is soft. Reduce heat. Dilute the kuzu in a little water. Add this to the fruit, stirring constantly to prevent it forming lumps. Simmer for 2–3 minutes or until thickened. Place in individual serving bowls. Garnish with mint leaves.

You can substitute the apples and pears of this recipe with any other seasonal fruit – plums, apricots or prunes.

100 g raisins

1 litre water

2 apples, washed and sliced

2 pears, washed and sliced

5-6 tbsp kuzu (a non-flavoured white root starch available from health food stores and Japanese supermarkets)

mint leaves, to garnish

SERVES 2

— STEWED PLUMS WITH CRUNCH —

PLACE plums, raisins, water and maple syrup (or barley malt) in a pan over a medium heat. Bring to the boil. Cover and simmer on low heat for 5–8 minutes. Meanwhile preheat oven to 180°C/350°F/Gas Mark 4. Dilute the kuzu in two tablespoons of water and add to the plums, stirring constantly. Simmer for 2–3 minutes. Pour this mix into a baking dish. Roast the oats in a dry skillet until golden. Place in a mixing bowl. Roast the rest of the nuts lightly before combining with the rice syrup. Sprinkle the nuts and seeds and the oats evenly to cover the plums. Serve warm.

12 plums, halved and pitted

100 g raisins

300 ml water

4 tbsp maple syrup or barley malt

2 tbsp kuzu

For the topping:

225 g rolled oats

4 tbsp walnuts

4 tbsp almonds

4 tbsp sunflower seeds

2 tbsp rice syrup

SERVES 2

— CARROT MACAROONS —

225 g raw carrots, grated
4 tbsp water
150 ml maple syrup or honey
2 tbsp sunflower oil
1 tsp almond extract
½ tsp vanilla extract
450 g dry and grated coconut
100 g wholewheat flour

SERVES 2

PREHEAT the oven to 180°C/350°F/Gas Mark 4. Oil a baking tray. Mix all the ingredients together in a bowl. Allow to sit for 15 minutes. Make macaroon shapes and place on baking sheet. Bake for 20–25 minutes until lightly browned.

— BANANA AND DATE COOKIES —

1½ bananas, mashed
225 g dates, chopped
450 g rolled oats
100 g almonds, chopped
4 tbsp oil
1 tsp vanilla extract

SERVES 2

PREHEAT the oven to 180°C/350°F/Gas Mark 4. Oil a baking tray. Mix all the ingredients well in a bowl and leave to rest for 10 minutes. Make cookie shapes and place them on the tray. Bake for 25 minutes until lightly browned.

FRUIT JUICE COCKTAILS

THE *best way of maximising the benefits from fresh juices is to incorporate them into your daily diet. Fresh fruit and vegetable juices are packed with natural vitamins, minerals and other supplements, as opposed to the synthetic variety that come in pill form. The body does not need to make an effort to absorb these natural supplements, whereas with the man-made variety they still need to be broken down in order to penetrate the bloodstream. A blood and immune booster which reduces blood toxicity levels and improves the immune system consists of integrating menus from our book with three 200 ml*

glasses of fresh juice a day; you will see the results within the first two weeks of this healthy regimen. If you want to restore your health and maintain a simple, effective and yet not drastic regimen, try drinking at least one glass of fresh juice every day and switch from your normal diet to meals taken from our recipes over several weeks or months – this will progressively build up your health.

We suggest that you drink fresh juices in the morning on an empty stomach as all the health properties in the juice will be easily absorbed into the bloodstream and you will obtain the maximum benefit. You can follow with a fruit breakfast from our breakfast menus; if you eat toast, croissants or bread with your juice, the bread will soak up the juice in your stomach and you may feel bloated. Leave a gap of 20 minutes between one item and the other or try eating a bowl of cereal with non-dairy milk instead. Fresh juices can be drunk all day long; they make great energy-boosters after a work-out or in mid- to late afternoon when the energy levels sink after a day of hard work. They are also very good when you are feeling ill and not very hungry – they give you all the nutrients without overworking your digestive system; in this case, serve them at room temperature, not chilled, but always freshly made.

There are infinite combinations of fruit and vegetable juices – here we give but a few suggestions that work for us. Explore with your own juice combinations and make up cocktails choosing fruit and vegetables that are in season. There are several books published with many recipes for juices that you might like to experiment with.

— CARROT AND CELERY JUICE —

*5 carrots per glass, washed and
ends chopped off
4 celery sticks per glass, washed*

CARROT is the king of all vegetable juices. It contains pro-vitamin A (which the body converts into vitamin A), vitamins B, C, D, E and K, as well as the minerals calcium, phosphorus, potassium, sodium and trace minerals. It cleanses the lining of the colon and intestines and it is one of the most naturally perfect cleansers and tonics for the liver. Through regular use, carrot juice helps the liver release excess bile and stale fats; when fat levels are reduced, cholesterol is also reduced.

Celery has a calming effect on the nervous system and it is a rich source of organic sodium – natural salt, which is less harmful than inorganic table salt as it naturally combines with many other minerals (the salty taste of our blood is due to it being high in organic sodium). In weight-reduction diets, celery juice helps reduce cravings for sweets.

— WATERMELON JUICE —

*Juice the entire fruit – rind, seeds and pulp – as it makes the
juice sweeter and adds many minerals contained in the rind.*

THIS is a great kidney and bladder cleanser and helps regulate excess fluids in the body. It stimulates the appetite and contains plenty of enzymes. In hot summer days, it can be drunk very cold throughout the day.

— APPLE AND PINEAPPLE JUICE —

*Skin the pineapple and use the flesh only – ⅙ of the fruit per
glass.
Use unpeeled firm apples of any variety – Golden Delicious,
Granny Smith, Pippin, Macintosh – whatever is available at
your local greengrocer, but make sure that they are not sprayed or
waxed; 2 to 3 apples per glass, depending on size.*

FRESH pineapple juice is sweet, thirst-quenching and very delicious when combined with apple. Pineapple juice is rich in vitamin C, enzymes and fruit acids and it soothes sore throats. It also contains bromelin which helps neutralise foods that are either too alkaline or too acidic and thus helps with indigestion.

Apple juice is rich in vitamins A, B1, B2, B6, C, biotin, folic acid, pantothenic acid and the minerals chlorine, copper, iron, magnesium, manganese, phosphorus, potassium, silicon, sodium and sulphur. The fresh vitamin C in apple juice helps prevent colds, flu and intestinal infections. Its high pectin content also makes it an excellent natural bowel regulator.

— BEETROOT, CARROT AND CELERY JUICE —

Choose uncooked beets, peeled – 1½ per glass
Carrots, unpeeled and washed – 5 or 6 per glass, depending on size
Celery sticks, washed – 3 or 4 per glass, depending on size

BEETROOT juice is an excellent source of vitamin B6, choline organic sodium and potassium and natural sugars. Beetroot yields high-quality iron that helps build red blood cells and is easily and effectively absorbed into the bloodstream. This is an excellent juice for winter when we need to build strength and keep our blood fluid to maintain good circulation. It is also very good for anaemia and for women to drink during their menstrual cycle. Beetroots are powerful kidney cleansers, so we suggest you use ¼ beets to ¾ carrots and celery, building up slowly to ½ beetroot and ½ carrots and celery. This is a powerful cocktail.

— ORANGE AND GRAPEFRUIT —

Pink and red grapefruits are sweeter and less acidic than the white variety. Peel them, quarter them and discard the seeds — use 1½ fruits per glass.
Use fresh whole oranges and not bottled orange juice — 1½ fruits per glass.

THIS combination makes a powerful tonic and cleanser for the gastro-intestinal tract. It also improves and strengthens capillary walls, benefiting the heart and lungs. Orange juice contains large amounts of vitamin A and C as well as minerals, bioflavonoids, amino acids and folic acid.

Grapefruit juice is also a rich source of vitamin C. This combination is excellent for treating common colds and sore throats. Grapefruit juice, for instance, will produce a light sweat and relieve fever.

— PINEAPPLE, APPLE, PEAR, STRAWBERRY AND RASPBERRY —

Use just a few raspberries, 5 or 6 per glass
Use between 6 and 8 strawberries per glass, depending on size
⅙ of pineapple per glass
1½ apples per glass
1 pear per glass

THIS is a delicious fruit cocktail, packed with vitamins. The pear makes for a thicker consistency, so that it resembles a smoothie more than a very liquid juice. The perfect drink for late spring and early summer.

NON-DAIRY FRUIT SMOOTHIES

FRUIT *smoothies are highly nutritious and a healthy substitute beverage for the mid-morning or mid-afternoon coffee or tea ritual. They can be made and drunk in all seasons. If at lunch-time you are not feeling overly hungry or are short of time, drink a smoothie instead as they are packed with all the necessary vitamins and nutrients. They are also great after your work-out at the health club. We suggest that you drink smoothies on their own, away from other food, as they represent a complete meal in themselves.*

• *Frozen bananas provide the creamy texture to all non-dairy fruit smoothies. Place unpeeled bananas in the freezer overnight. When ready to prepare the smoothie, allow bananas to thaw for 30 minutes before putting them into the blender.*

• *Use natural sweeteners such as unheated raw honey organic maple syrup or blended dates.*

• *If frozen fruits don't suit your digestion, use fruits at room temperature and combine in the blender with fruit juices which have been frozen beforehand.*

• *Fresh or dried coconut adds creamy texture to smoothies.*

— BANANA, DATE AND APPLE SMOOTHIE —

THE day before, freeze the bananas and the apple juice overnight. Allow fruit to thaw for 30 minutes before preparing the smoothie. Place all the ingredients in a blender and blend well. You can dilute with more apple juice or a little soy milk.

2 bananas per glass
1½ apples per glass – choose organic apples, Granny Smith, Golden Delicious or the season's variety – juiced
6 dates per glass

— BANANA, STRAWBERRY AND PINEAPPLE JUICE —

⅙ pineapple per glass, juiced and frozen

2 bananas per glass, frozen

6 or 7 strawberries per glass, frozen

ALLOW fruit to thaw for 30 minutes before placing in a blender to combine thoroughly.

— PAPAYA, BANANA AND COCONUT —

1 glass coconut milk, frozen

2 bananas per glass, frozen

½ papaya, frozen

ALLOW fruit to thaw for 30 minutes. Place in a blender and blend thoroughly.

— BANANA AND BLUEBERRIES WITH MAPLE SYRUP —

2 bananas per glass, frozen

10–15 blueberries per glass, frozen

3 tbsp maple syrup

ALLOW the bananas and the blueberries to thaw for 30 minutes. Place in blender with the maple syrup and blend thoroughly.

— FRESH WATERMELON AND CANTALOUPE SMOOTHIE —

1 watermelon, half the pulp frozen and the other half juiced and frozen

½ cantaloupe melon, frozen

ALLOW to thaw for 30 minutes. Put all the fruit ingredients in a blender and combine thoroughly.

Chapter 4

SPRING

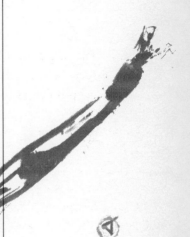

THE *equinox on March 21 marks the beginning of spring – the season of blossoms. From now on for the next six months* yang *energy progressively grows and is dominant in nature – everything is being born again. There is a marked increase in the amount of sunlight during the days, awakening us from the sleep of winter. The element of this season is wood. This is the perfect time for long walks in nature, where the sight of the surrounding green plants growing heals our bodies and nourishes our souls. Outdoor activities also help us to oxygenate after the long winter months; our appetite decreases and we get rid of winter fats.*

This is a time for fresh beginnings, new resolutions and looking at life and its mysteries with new cleansed eyes – Chinese medicine says that spring strips off the invisible membrane over our eyes and minds and gives a clearer picture. Now is the time to bring positive energy into old, destructive patterns, renew friendships and re-value all those relationships and activities which bring us joy, wholeness and fulfilment.

To keep pace with this new brighter and lighter phase we eat foods that promote the taste for this season – sour. This is the season where we eat less or even fast to cleanse our bodies from the excesses of autumn and winter and pay special attention to the liver and gall bladder.

— SPRING COOKING METHODS —

Steaming raw food and quick cooking at high temperatures such as stir-frying.

— SPRING FOODS —

Green beans, peppers, all manner of young plants, new potatoes, baby asparagus, sprouts, cereal grasses (wheat), young beets, carrots, starchy vegetables, lemons and salads.

— SPRING GRAINS —

Quinoa, barley, rye, oats and sprouted grains.

— SPRING FRUITS —

Apples and pears.

— SPECIAL FOODS —

Emphasise fermented foods like tempeh, sauerkraut and live yoghurt.

— SPRING HERBS —

Basil, caraway, parsley, dill, bay leaf. Also raw onion and garlic help with spring digestion.

— SUGGESTED BODY THERAPIES —

All therapies in spring should be aimed at cleansing and renewal – long walks in nature, in forests and by the side of water to oxygenate the lungs. Also open-air activities such as gardening or *tai chi* in the park. To help cleansing, eat raw food, drink fresh juices and take a course in colonic irrigation.

— SUGGESTED DIET —

Salads, *sushi,* lightly steamed vegetables, stir-fries, sandwiches, light seasonings, use less oil on your meals. Also moderate the use of vinegar and lemons.

LUNCH

All recipes serve between 4–6

— TEMPEH SANDWICHES —

HEAT the oil in a frying pan. Add garlic and tempeh and continue to fry until browned evenly on both sides. When almost ready, add tamari sauce to tempeh. To assemble the sandwich: lightly toast the bread and spread the Russian dressing on all the bread slices. Take three slices and evenly distribute watercress on each, placing on top a slice of tempeh. Top it with onion and tomato rings. Put another slice of bread on top and serve with dill pickle or wrap them well for later.

4 tbsp sunflower oil
1 garlic clove, chopped
225 g tempeh, thinly sliced
2 tbsp tamari sauce
4–6 slices rye bread
300 ml Tofu Russian dressing
(see recipe on page 43)
225 g watercress or alfalfa
sprouts
onion rings or chopped spring
onions
1 large tomato, thinly sliced
dill pickle (optional)

MAKES 2 TO 3 SANDWICHES

– LENTIL BURGERS –

225 g green lentils, washed
900 ml stock
1 bay leaf
1 pinch each sea salt and pepper
4 tbsp extra-virgin olive oil
1 onion, chopped
1 garlic clove, chopped
350 g mushrooms, finely chopped
2 tbsp tomato purée
finely chopped fresh parsley
100 g breadcrumbs
4 tbsp wholewheat flour, seasoned
with herbs

PUT the lentils, bay leaf, vegetable stock and seasonings over a medium heat. Cover and cook for 45 minutes to 1 hour.

When lentils are tender, remove from heat, drain and mash them coarsely with a potato masher. Heat two tablespoons of oil and sauté onion and garlic until lightly browned. Next add mushrooms, stir well and cook them for 2–4 minutes.

Remove from the pan and add mushroom mix to lentils along with tomato purée and parsley. Adjust seasoning. Add the breadcrumbs.

From this mix make small flat cakes and leave them to rest for 30 minutes. Coat the burgers with seasoned flour. Heat remaining oil and fry the burgers evenly on both sides on low medium heat. For a low-fat alternative, the burgers can be grilled until brown on both sides. Serve them hot with tomato and cucumber rings and a savoury dip.

– BARLEY AND HAZELNUT SALAD –

225 g uncooked barley
700 ml stock
4 tbsp olive oil
2 celery sticks, chopped
225 g carrots, finely chopped
225 g hazelnuts, finely chopped
4 tbsp chopped fresh parsley
4 tbsp currants, soaked in
hot water
100 g toasted hazelnuts

RINSE the barley well. Add stock to it and bring to the boil. Lower heat and simmer until all the water is absorbed. Allow to cool.

When barley is cool, add rest of the ingredients and toss with the vinaigrette dressing (see opposite). Season with salt and pepper.

WHISK all ingredients together and add to the barley salad.

For the vinaigrette:
2 tbsp hazelnut oil
4 tsp lemon juice
1 tsp wine vinegar
2 spring onions, finely chopped
1 clove garlic, chopped
2 tbsp orange juice

— BAKED TOFU AND CURLY ENDIVE PLATTER —

TO marinate the tofu: drain and press for 15 minutes to get rid of excess water. Cut into 2.5 cm chunks.

In a bowl, combine three garlic cloves with the tomato purée, sherry vinegar and tamari sauce and two tablespoons of water. Whisk well, add tofu chunks and mix well. Cover and refrigerate for 30 minutes. Toss 2 to 3 times while in the refrigerator.

Heat oil in a frying pan and sauté onion, sprinkling with the oregano until soft. Next add mushrooms with the remaining garlic clove. Fry until mushrooms are soft, sprinkle with sesame seeds.

Put the grill on a medium heat. Mix the tofu with breadcrumbs or corn flour and place under the grill. Brown the tofu evenly on all sides, turning every 6 minutes. (Can be done while mushrooms cool.) Toss mushroom and tofu mix together and serve over endive leaves which have been sprinkled with oil beforehand.

1 block tofu (marinated overnight)
4 garlic cloves, chopped
2 tbsp tomato purée
4 tsp sherry vinegar
3 tbsp tamari sauce
2 tbsp sesame oil
1 medium red onion, sliced
1 pinch dried oregano
450 g mushrooms, sliced
3 tsp black sesame seeds, toasted
breadcrumbs or corn flour
curly endive

— BUTTER BEAN BRUSCHETTA WITH GARLIC MUSTARD GREENS —

2 tbsp olive oil
1 small onion, chopped
1 tsp dried thyme and sage
1 pinch each sea salt and pepper
2 garlic cloves, chopped
1 celery stick, chopped
375 g cooked butter beans or
haricot beans
1 tbsp tomato purée
1 tsp cider vinegar
450 g chopped and steamed
mustard greens
chopped tomatoes
4 slices country bread, cut into
2.5 cm pieces

HEAT half the olive oil on a medium heat. Add onion together with thyme, sage and a pinch of salt. Cook until slightly soft. Add half the garlic and celery. Sauté until transparent.

Add beans together with tomato purée and vinegar. Mix well and crush beans with the back of a wooden spoon as they cook. Place this mix in a blender and blend until smooth. Drizzle with extra oil. Adjust seasonings. In another frying pan, heat oil, add the other half of the garlic and mustard greens and stir to coat evenly with oil. Sprinkle with salt, pepper and chopped tomatoes. Set aside.

To assemble: toast the bread lightly. Mound the bean purée on the bread and top with greens.

DINNER

All recipes serve between 4–6

STARTERS

— SPINACH AND CHICKPEA SOUP WITH CUMIN CROÛTONS —

WARM three tablespoons of oil in a soup pot, add onion, garlic and salt. Sauté briefly before adding cumin, nutmeg, cloves and bay leaf. Cook and stir briefly, adding extra oil if necessary. Add cooked chickpeas and 600 ml of stock. Simmer for 10 minutes. Add spinach leaves to the pot and allow them to wilt. Add remaining stock. Bring to the boil and simmer for 10–15 minutes to let the chickpeas absorb the flavour. Cool the soup briefly, then purée in a blender. Return to the pot, season with lemon juice, salt and pepper. If necessary thin the soup.

4 tbsp extra-virgin olive oil

1 red onion, diced

3 garlic cloves, chopped

1 pinch each sea salt and pepper

1 tsp cumin powder

¼ tsp nutmeg

1 bay leaf

2 cloves

325 g cooked chickpeas (save the cooking liquid)

1 litre 900 ml Curry Stock (see page 58)

900 g chopped spinach leaves

1 tbsp lemon juice

BEAT the egg white until frothy, add all the remaining ingredients except bread cubes and blend. Toss bread cubes in egg white mix and bake evenly in an oiled tray at 190°C/375°F/Gas Mark 5 for 10 minutes.

For the cumin croûtons:

1 egg white

1 tsp chopped garlic

2 tsp ground cumin

½ tsp salt

2 tsp chopped coriander

225 g small bread cubes

— STUFFED COURGETTES WITH OLIVE AND TOMATO MARINADE —

3 medium courgettes
1 fresh thyme sprig
2 tbsp extra-virgin olive oil
1 large onion, chopped
2 garlic cloves, chopped
1 tbsp each chopped fresh basil
and parsley
2 firm tomatoes, skinned, seeded
and chopped
4 tbsp wholewheat breadcrumbs
4 tbsp ground walnuts

PREHEAT oven to 190°C/375°F/Gas Mark 5. Oil a large baking tray. Wash the courgettes, cut them in half lengthways and remove the pulp with a spoon. Chop the pulp and save it. Steam the courgette halves over salted boiling water with a sprig of thyme for 6–8 minutes – soft but not too tender. Remove and let them cool on the oiled baking tray. In the meantime, heat oil in a frying pan, add onion, garlic and salt. Sauté until lightly browned. Add basil, parsley and the chopped courgette pulp, mix well and cook for a further 2 minutes. Add the tomato flesh. Adjust seasonings. Remove from heat and mix in the crumbs and walnuts, blending well. Fill courgettes with the stuffing, drizzling some olive oil on top. Place them in a preheated oven for 15–20 minutes. Then brown the top under a grill. Serve hot with olive and tomato marinade (see below).

For the marinade:
4 tbsp olive paste
4 tbsp tomato purée

MIX the olive and tomato purée well, add a little water and warm lightly before serving.

— ASPARAGUS ORIENTAL-STYLE —

450 g asparagus
2 tsp sesame oil
1 leek, thinly sliced like
matchsticks
1 tbsp chopped root ginger
2 garlic cloves, chopped
4 tbsp water
toasted sesame seeds, to sprinkle
For the marinade:
2 tbsp tamari sauce
½ tsp honey
1 tbsp sherry
2 tsp cornstarch + 1 tbsp water
1 tbsp sesame oil

COMBINE marinade ingredients and set aside. Trim and wash the asparagus, removing tough ends. Heat the oil in a wok. When hot, add leek. Sauté for 2 minutes. Add garlic and ginger. Stir for a few seconds. Add asparagus. Stir once more, adding the water. Simmer for 5 minutes until the vegetables are tender.

Whisk the marinade and pour it over the vegetables in the wok. Turn the heat to high. Stir for 1 minute until the sauce thickens. Serve warm with a sprinkling of sesame seeds.

— CAULIFLOWER SOUFFLÉ —

Trim the cauliflower and cut into large pieces and steam for 20 to 30 minutes. Drain and break cauliflower into small pieces.

Heat oil in a wok, mix in the cauliflower and stir well. Let all the florets get coated with oil. Combine soaked bread with cauliflower in a blender and purée the mixture. Return the purée to heat and warm through, adjusting the seasonings.

Preheat the oven to 200°C/400°F/Gas mark 6. Oil the soufflé pan liberally and sprinkle with breadcrumbs. Pour the cauliflower mix into prepared pan and bake in the oven for 15 minutes until brown on top. Serve with parsley and walnut sauce (below).

HEAT the stock with the parsley and the walnuts. When hot, add soy cream and stir well.

1 large cauliflower
2 tbsp olive oil
4 slices wholewheat bread soaked in milk for 15 minutes
1 garlic clove, chopped
2 tbsp breadcrumbs
1 tsp chopped fresh herbs such as parsley, rosemary
salt, pepper, mustard

For the parsley and walnut sauce:
150 ml stock
225 g fresh parsley, finely chopped
4 tbsp walnuts, chopped and toasted
4 tbsp soy cream

— ARTICHOKE CROSTINI —

ARRANGE the bread slices on a baking tray, brush each one with olive oil on both sides and toast lightly. Mix the black olive paste with garlic and a few drops of olive oil. Spread the paste on each slice after it is toasted. Top with a slice of tomato, arrange slices of artichoke on top, drizzle olive oil and grill briefly. Sprinkle with basil and serve right away.

1 good quality baguette, sliced into 1 cm thick slices
2 tbsp olive oil
4 tbsp black olive paste
2 small garlic cloves, mashed
1 small red tomato, sliced thinly
8 marinated artichokes, cut into quarters lengthways
6 fresh basil leaves

MAIN MEALS

— BLACK BEAN STEW WITH GRILLED POLENTA AND APPLE AND RAISIN SAUCE —

325 g black beans, soaked
overnight
1 litre 600 ml water
1 bay leaf
3 tsp cumin seeds
1 tsp each chopped fresh basil
and oregano
2 tbsp oil
2 medium onions, chopped
3 garlic cloves, chopped
2 celery sticks, chopped
1½ tsp ground coriander
1 pinch paprika
1 carrot, diced
1 medium yellow pepper, chopped
325 g tomatoes, blanched in hot
water, skinned and chopped
1 tbsp rice vinegar
4 tbsp chopped coriander
1 pinch each sea salt and pepper

WASH and drain the beans well. Cover them with fresh water and salt and bring to the boil with a bay leaf. Cover and simmer until tender for about 1–1½ hours. Meanwhile, prepare rest of the recipe.

Heat half the oil over a medium heat. Add cumin seeds and when they begin to colour, add oregano and basil. Keep stirring to prevent herbs from scorching, adding extra oil if necessary. Add onion and garlic and salt together with coriander and paprika and cook for 15 minutes. Add carrot and yellow pepper. Mix well and cook for 5 minutes or so before adding the tomatoes. Mix all ingredients well with the tomatoes and let them simmer for 10–12 minutes. If the mixture gets dry, add a little water.

Test the beans, if done – drain in a colander, saving 150 ml of cooking liquid. Add the drained beans to the tomato mix. Stir well and let the flavours soak in as it cooks for ½ hour. When needed, add bean liquid to prevent the mix becoming too dry. Test for seasonings and tenderness of beans. When ready garnish with vinegar, coriander and Sour Cream (see page 41).

For the grilled polenta:
1 litre 300 ml water
1 tsp each sea salt and pepper
325 g coarse maize meal
2 tbsp extra-virgin olive oil

BRING the water to the boil, add salt and pepper, then pour the corn meal in a thin stream, stirring constantly with a wooden spoon, so as to avoid the formation of any lumps. Reduce the heat and cook, stirring constantly, for 30 minutes or cook in a double broiler for 45 minutes. Oil a baking dish and pour the cooked polenta into it. Set aside to cool and firm. When cool, cut it into 1 cm slices, brush them with olive oil and grill them until browned.

In a saucepan cook the apples with the cider and the maple syrup for 8–10 minutes until tender. Stir in the soaked raisins and all the spices. Cook for another 2 minutes and serve as the sauce.

For the apple and raisin sauce:
300 ml warm apple cider
450 g green apples, peeled and diced
2 tbsp maple syrup
175 g raisins, soaked in warm water
½ tsp allspice
½ cinnamon powder
1 tsp each sea salt and cayenne pepper

— SUSHI WITH GREEN BEAN SALAD AND GINGER TOFU —

Rinse the rice well or until the water is clear. Leave to drain. Place rice and water in a pan and cook covered over a medium heat for 10–12 minutes. Reduce heat to low and cook until the water is fully absorbed. Remove from heat and allow it to stand covered for 10 minutes.

Heat the vinegar, mirin and salt over a low heat until the salt is dissolved. Put the rice in a large bowl and fan it vigorously to cool it. Slowly stir in the mirin and vinegar mix. Continue fanning and stirring until cool.

Scoop out the seeds from the cucumber and cut in 1 cm strips. Place a sheet of toasted nori on a bamboo rolling mat and with damp hands cover it with a layer of rice. Spread a thin line of wasabi across the rice from left to right. Place 1 cm line of cucumber strips over wasabi using bamboo roller. Roll the sushi away from you with a sharp wet knife and cut into 2.5 cm pieces. Serve with ginger and tamari sauce.

For the sushi:
225 g Japanese white rice
450 ml cups water
2 tbsp rice vinegar
4 tbsp mirin
½ tsp salt
1 medium cucumber, peeled and cut lengthways
4 sheets nori, toasted
1 tbsp wasabi, dissolved in water
pickled ginger and tamari sauce, to serve

For the green bean salad:
450 g green beans, stringed and
cut into 5 cm lengths
4 tbsp miso
toasted sesame seeds
1 tbsp mirin
1 tbsp sugar

COOK the beans in boiling water until tender. Rinse under cold water. Make dressing by mixing miso with sesame seeds. Add mirin and sugar. Combine this dressing with the cooked beans until they are well covered. Leave it to rest for 15 minutes before serving.

For the ginger tofu:
250 g fresh tofu
4 tbsp cornflour
2 tbsp vegetable oil
2.5 cm piece fresh root ginger, cut
into matchsticks
2 leeks, washed and sliced
4 tbsp tamari sauce
1 tbsp mirin
1 tbsp sugar
200 ml water
4 spring onions, sliced diagonally
½ cup beansprouts

WRAP the tofu in a clean towel for about 30 minutes until all the excess water has been drained, then cut into cubes and dust with cornflour.

Heat half the oil in a skillet and sauté the tofu cubes, stirring often until evenly brown. Drain on a kitchen towel.

Heat the remaining oil and sauté leeks and ginger for 2–3 minutes. Add remaining ingredients (except for beansprouts and spring onions) and sauté for a further 3–4 minutes, stirring all the time. Lastly, add the cubed tofu, mixing well and sautéing for another 2–3 minutes. Serve hot and sprinkle with beansprouts and spring onions.

— MEDITERRANEAN TIAM WITH GREEK SALAD —

PREHEAT the oven to 200°C/400°F/Gas Mark 6. Oil a round or square baking dish. Heat the oil in a frying pan and sauté onions and garlic briefly. In the oiled baking dish, layer up courgettes, onions and tomatoes. Repeat until you have 2–3 layers of each. Finish on top with tomatoes. Season and sprinkle with chopped basil. Combine vegetable stock, tomato purée and pesto and pour evenly over the vegetable tiam. Cover with foil and cook in preheated oven for 45 minutes.

Combine breadcrumbs and parsley; remove the foil cover from the vegetable casserole and spread the bread-crumb mix over the layer of tomatoes and brown under a grill for 5 minutes. Serve hot or at room temperature.

For the tiam:
2 tbsp sunflower oil
2 onions, sliced
2 garlic cloves, crushed
4 courgettes sliced, salted and drained
4 tomatoes, sliced
2 tbsp fresh chopped basil
4 tbsp vegetable stock
1 tbsp tomato purée
1 tsp ready-made pesto
3 tbsp breadcrumbs
2 tbsp each fresh chopped parsley, celery, onions
1 pinch each sea salt and pepper

TOSS all the ingredients together and combine with a dressing of your choice.

For the Greek salad:
1 head romaine lettuce, washed and torn into bite-size pieces
a few leaves of baby spinach or arugula
a few Greek olives
1 red and 1 yellow pepper, cut into thin strips
1 red onion, thinly sliced
a few sun-dried tomatoes, chopped
a few pieces feta cheese or tofu or bread croûtons
1/2 avocado, thinly sliced
1/2 cucumber, thinly sliced
1 celery stick, thinly sliced

— TOFU AND VEGETABLE KEBABS WITH SAFFRON AND CARDAMOM RICE —

1 green and 1 yellow pepper, cut
into pieces
8 shallots, peeled and kept whole
8 baby squash or courgettes
30 g tofu, cut into 12 pieces
8 mushrooms, wiped clean
bamboo skewers, soaked in water

For the marinade:
3 tbsp soy sauce
1 tbsp tomato purée
2 garlic cloves, crushed
1 tbsp sugar
1 tsp balsamic vinegar
4 tbsp olive oil

MIX together all the marinade ingredients well.

Thread the vegetables onto bamboo skewers. Brush all sides with the marinade and place them in a deep oven-proof dish. Pour the leftover marinade over the vegetables and leave to marinate for 4–6 hours (min. 2 hours).

Just before dinner, grill the vegetables, brushing with marinade as you turn them to get them evenly cooked. Grill for 5–7 minutes. Serve on a bed of rice, following the recipe below.

Saffron and Cardamom Rice:
225 g basmati rice
1 tbsp sunflower oil
2 whole cardamom pods, crushed
1 cm stick cinnamon
600 ml water
1 pinch sea salt
¼ tsp saffron threads, dissolved
in 2 tbsp warm water
1 tbsp sultanas, soaked in
hot water

WASH the rice in several changes of water and leave to soak for 30 minutes. Heat oil in a rice pot, stir in crushed cardamom and cinnamon. Fry for 1–2 minutes. Add drained rice and fry for another 3 minutes on a low heat. Add the water and salt. Bring to the boil, reduce heat and let it simmer until all the water is absorbed.

Stir in saffron and sultanas just as rice is ready to be served. Mix and fluff the rice well. Rice can be kept warm in the oven at a moderate heat.

— PASTA PRIMAVERA —

PREHEAT the grill to a high temperature, put the peppers on a baking sheet and cook, turning often until surfaces are charred. Transfer peppers to an airtight bag or sealed container to cool.

When cool, peel the skin from the peppers. Split each pepper into half and remove seeds and ribs, but save the juices. Purée the peppers.

Heat oil in a pan, add onion and garlic, followed by leeks, chard and the peas. Stir fry at a low heat. Add salt and pepper. When vegetables are done, add purée of red pepper, spring onions and Japanese five-spice mix. Cook or warm briefly.

Cook pasta as per instructions on the packet in salted boiling water. Drain and mix well with vegetable sauce. Sprinkle with toasted pine nuts and basil leaves.

450 g soba noodles (or tagliatelle or spinach fettuccine)

3 red peppers

4 tbsp extra-virgin olive oil

1 red onion, sliced

2 garlic cloves, chopped

2 leeks, finely chopped

325 g Swiss chard, cut into strips

450 g peas

6 tbsp spring onions, chopped

½ tsp Japanese five-spice powder

2 tbsp pine nuts

6 or 8 fresh basil leaves, cut into strips

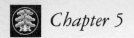

Chapter 5

MIDSUMMER

IN *summer* yang *energy is at its height in nature —*
everything is ripening and bearing fruit. To unify with
this beautiful season we will express expansion, growth,
lightness, outward activity and creativity. June 21 sets
the beginning of summer, when days are longer and
nights shorter — this is the time for outdoor activities,
like swimming at the seaside or the lakes with long
hours spent in contact with nature wearing little cloth-
ing, safely exposing the skin to the warm rays of the sun.

Everywhere around us is a symphony of colours and
our summer tables should carry dazzling displays of the
abundant produce available now. This is the time for
informal eating and great get-togethers with family and
friends — picnics, outdoor barbecues, eating in the garden
or patio.

In summer we must pay particular attention to bal-
ance the taking of our meals with the heat. So eat plenty
of cooling foods at room temperature (icy cold drinks and
ice creams can contract our digestive systems), drink
plenty of liquids and try eating when the sun is not at
its hottest (lunch should be later than normal and din-
ner should be well after sunset). Try to create a cool
atmosphere by closing shutters early in the morning to
trap the fresh air, using light cotton sheets on beds and
watering your plants and garden frequently.

— SUMMER COOKING METHODS —

Raw foods, light steaming, cooking at high heats for short times, such as stir-frying.

— SUMMER FOODS —

Green leafy bitter vegetables, lettuce, endive, watercress, cucumbers, cabbage, alfalfa, corn, mushrooms, beansprouts, spring onions.

— SUMMER GRAINS —

Rolled oats, lentils, millet, yellow corn.

— SUMMER FRUITS —

Strawberries, apricots, cherries, red plums, peaches.

— SUMMER DRINKING LIQUIDS —

Preferably at room temperature; lemonade, occasionally sprinkled with ginger, cold teas, especially fruity teas such as strawberry and fruit and vegetable juices.

— SUMMER HERBS —

Mint, chrysanthemum, horseradish.

— SUGGESTED BODY THERAPIES —

Swimming, scuba-diving, jogging, tennis and outdoor ball games. Colour therapy, outdoor yoga and *tai chi*.

— SUGGESTED DIET —

Very light meals, preferably taken often in small quantities, emphasising lunch as the main meal. Crisp salads, cold udon noodles with tofu, corn on the cob, raw vegetables with a dressing, fruit salads.

LUNCH

— EASY TOFU BURGERS —

1 tbsp extra-virgin olive oil
100 g chopped spring onions
450 g grated cabbage
450 g shredded carrots
225 g firm tofu, drained
2 tbsp soy sauce
2 tsp baking powder
seasonings: oregano, paprika, ginger
100 g wholewheat flour
wholewheat buns, to serve

For the salad:
1 tomato, sliced
alfalfa
dill pickle
soy mayonnaise
½ cucumber, sliced

PREHEAT oven to 180°C/350°F Gas Mark 4. Heat oil in a skillet, add onions, cabbage and carrot. Stir well and sauté for 4–5 minutes until slightly tender.

Cream the tofu in a blender, add soy sauce, baking powder and seasonings. Blend well. Put the creamed tofu in a bowl and mix with sautéed vegetables. Test for seasonings.

Make flat patties from this mixture, dust them with flour and place them on an oiled baking sheet. Bake for 15 minutes, turn over and bake for an additional 10 minutes. The burgers can also be grilled until brown.

Serve tofu burgers in a wholewheat bun with the salad.

— SALAD OF GRILLED SUMMER VEGETABLES —

HEAT the grill. Combine all sliced vegetables in a bowl with olive oil, balsamic vinegar and seasonings. Toss well, so all vegetables have a coating of oil. Place these vegetables on an oiled rack under the grill about 10 cm from the heat. Brush them with oil if they become dry. Turn them over and grill 5 minutes on each side until lightly browned.

Transfer the grilled vegetables onto a serving platter and drizzle with more olive oil, sprinkling with fresh basil and parsley.

1 large onion, cut into slices
1 large courgette, cut into
diagonal slices
2 yellow squash, cut into 1 cm
diagonal slices
2 large carrots, sliced diagonally
1 red and 1 green pepper, cut into
squares
4 tbsp extra-virgin olive oil
2 tbsp balsamic vinegar
1 pinch each sea salt and pepper
chopped fresh basil/parsley, to
garnish

— SPROUTED LENTIL SALAD —

BLEND all dressing ingredients in a food processor until creamy and pour into a large salad bowl. Add lentils and salad ingredients to the bowl with dressing. Toss well. Refrigerate until ready to serve.

450 g sprouted lentils (or
chickpea or mung bean sprouts)
100 g chopped tomatoes
4 tbsp pitted olives
4 tbsp sliced celery
4 tbsp chopped spring onions
4 tbsp finely chopped yellow or red
pepper
4 tbsp chopped fresh parsley
100 g alfalfa

For the dressing:
2 tbsp olive oil
¼ tsp ground cumin
½ tomato
¼ cucumber, peeled
100 g soaked sunflower seeds
1 pinch each sea salt and pepper

— CHICKPEA AND APPLE SALAD —

2 tbsp soy flour
300 ml dry cider
4 tbsp olive oil
4 tbsp cider vinegar
675 g cooked chickpeas
3 celery sticks, chopped
2 large eating apples, chopped (at
the last moment to prevent them
from turning brown)
100 g raisins, soaked in warm
water
chopped fresh coriander
pitta bread, to serve

STIR the soy flour with the cider in a saucepan. Set the pan on a low heat and bring the mix to the boil. Simmer for 15 minutes, stirring often. Take the sauce off the heat and let it cool. When cool, whisk in oil and vinegar.

In a bowl mix together the chickpeas, chopped celery, apples and raisins. Pour the cider sauce over the salad and toss well. Sprinkle with coriander. Serve with warm pitta bread.

— ROASTED RED PEPPER AND WATERCRESS SANDWICHES —

4 slices wholegrain bread, lightly
toasted
4 tbsp dairy-free mayonnaise
225 g watercress
3 red peppers, roasted, seeded
and sliced
1 carrot, grated
½ cucumber, thinly sliced
1 pinch each sea salt and pepper

SPREAD mayonnaise on the lightly toasted bread slices. Assemble the sandwich by adding watercress, pepper, grated carrots and cucumber in layers. Sprinkle with salt and pepper. Top with another slice of bread. Cut in triangles and serve with extra salad on the side.

DINNER

STARTERS

— BRAISED FENNEL —

TRIM the fennel ends and feathery fronds which can be used as a garnish. Remove any tough outer ribs. Halve and thinly slice the fennel lengthways.

    Heat oil in a pan. Toss in fennel, garlic and sesame seeds and cook, stirring all the time until slightly brown. Add half the lemon rind and the lemon juice along with vegetable stock. Bring to the boil, lower the heat and simmer gently for 15 minutes. Serve after seasoning with salt and pepper with the rest of the lemon rind.

2 large fennel bulbs
1 tbsp extra-virgin olive oil
2 garlic cloves, chopped
2 tbsp sesame seeds
6 tbsp vegetable stock (see page 58)
grated rind and juice of 1 lemon

— CHICORY AND BEAN SALAD —

PLACE the chicory in a salad bowl. Combine cooked beans with rest of the ingredients and salad dressing. Toss well. Add this bean mix over the bed of chicory salad. Serve extra salad dressing on the side.

450 g chicory or Belgian endive
375 g cooked white beans (navy beans are best for this recipe)
2 green peppers, diced small
4 spring onions, chopped
4 tbsp chopped fresh parsley
2 tbsp snipped chives
1 tsp chopped fresh thyme
8 black olives, pitted and chopped
2 large tomatoes, seeded and diced

For the dressing:
2–3 garlic cloves, chopped
2 tbsp mustard
4 tbsp wine vinegar
6 tbsp olive oil

— MUSTARD-LACED CUCUMBER SOUP —

4 large cucumbers, peeled, seeded
and cubed

3 spring onions, chopped

2 tsp chopped garlic

1 tsp chopped fresh root ginger

1 tsp each ground cumin and
coriander

1 pinch cinnamon powder

1 pinch each sea salt and pepper

2 tbsp chopped fresh mint

1 tbsp rice syrup

600 ml yoghurt, whisked

600 ml fresh carrot juice or
vegetable stock, chilled

2 tsp olive oil

2 tbsp mustard seeds

snipped fresh chives

COMBINE first nine ingredients well and chill them in a refrigerator from 30 minutes to 2 hours. Place this mix in a food processor and blend well. Place in a large bowl.

Whisk the cool yoghurt and carrot juice into the soup. Just before serving heat the oil and add mustard seeds. Cook stirring constantly until seeds pop. Pour this mix over the soup. Serve chilled with fresh chives sprinkled on top.

— ITALIAN BREAD SALAD —

900 g cubed wholewheat bread

1 small red onion, sliced

1 head lettuce, torn into bite-
sized pieces

225 g chopped peeled cucumber

225 g diced carrots

100 g chopped radishes

225 g cleaned, sliced mushrooms

4 spring onions, sliced

4 tbsp olives, pitted

2 tbsp capers

2 garlic cloves, chopped

2 tbsp chopped fresh parsley

5 tbsp extra-virgin olive oil

2 tbsp orange juice

3 tbsp balsamic vinegar

1 pinch each sea salt and pepper

SOAK the bread cubes in water for 30 minutes.

Soak the red onion slices in water for 40 minutes. In a bowl combine lettuce and all vegetables, including olives, capers, garlic and parsley.

Prepare salad dressing by mixing olive oil with vinegar orange juice, salt and pepper.

Drain onion, pat dry and add to salad bowl. Squeeze the water from the bread cubes and crumble them over the salad. Whisk the dressing and pour over the salad. Toss well and serve.

— AVOCADO SOUP —

HEAT the oil in a pan. Add onion, garlic and spring onions and sauté together with cumin and salt until soft but not brown.

Wash and drain the diced potatoes and add them to the frying pan. Mix well with onions and spices. Add the vegetable stock, cover and simmer for 15–20 minutes.

Peel the avocados, cut them into pieces and place in a blender together with the lime juice and purée until creamy.

When potatoes are soft, remove from heat and let them cool. When cool, transfer to the blender with avocado purée. Mix in the yoghurt and coriander. Blend well and check for seasonings.

Transfer the soup to a large glass bowl and add yoghurt to thin the consistency. Cover the soup and chill for 2 hours in the refrigerator before serving. Serve cool with chopped red pepper as garnish.

3 tbsp extra-virgin olive oil

100 g diced onions

2 garlic cloves, chopped

6 spring onions, chopped

1 pinch cumin

2 potatoes, diced in small cubes

900 ml vegetable stock

2 avocados

4 tbsp lime juice

300 ml soy yoghurt

2 tbsp chopped fresh coriander

2 tbsp chopped red pepper

MAIN MEALS

— GADO GADO —

3 carrots, sliced diagonally

250 g cauliflower florets

12 mangetouts, snipped and cut
in half

4 potatoes

tamari sauce

6 radishes, sliced

30 g tofu, drained and cubed

½ small cabbage, shredded

450 g mung bean sprouts

6 spring onions, chopped

chopped fresh coriander

rice crackers

STEAM the carrots, cauliflower and mangetouts briefly over the boiling potatoes. Drain potatoes; when done, run them under cold water and slice thinly.

Sprinkle a little tamari sauce over the tofu cubes and grill until slightly browned evenly on all sides and let them cool.

When vegetables are cool enough to handle, arrange them on individual plates, starting with the radishes and shredded cabbage in the middle and the potatoes arranged in a circle around the cabbage, alternating with the carrots and cauliflower. Arrange tofu cubes and mangetouts over the cabbage in the middle. Sprinkle with mung bean sprouts, spring onions and coriander evenly.

Serve this salad with tamari sauce on the side and rice crackers.

For the sauce:

2 tbsp vegetable oil

1 onion, finely chopped

3 garlic cloves, chopped

2 tsp chopped fresh root ginger

2 celery sticks, chopped

1 tbsp sugar

juice of 1 lemon

175 g crunchy peanut or other
nut butter

4 tbsp coconut milk

tamari sauce

¼ tsp cayenne

170 ml vegetable stock
(see page 58)

Making the sauce:

HEAT the oil, sauté onion, garlic and ginger, add celery and stir well. Cook until slightly brown. To the onion mix, add all the remaining ingredients and keep stirring over a low heat until the butter has completely melted. If it is too thick, add vegetable stock or hot water and adjust seasonings. Always serve the sauce warm.

— STUFFED TOMATOES WITH MAIZE AND PUMPKIN MEAL —

HEAT the oven to 160°C/325°F/Gas Mark 3. Oil a shallow oven-proof dish. Slice the tomatoes at the top and carefully scoop out the pulp and seeds. Save for later use. Cut a very thin slice from the bottoms so that the tomatoes can stand upright without toppling over.

Heat some oil in a pan and add onion, garlic and salt. Sauté for a few minutes and then add the cumin, coriander and pepper. Stir and cook for 4–5 minutes. Next add the cooked beans together with the flour mixture and vinegar and bay leaf. Mix well and cook on a low heat, stirring often. If it gets too dry, add a little of the tomato pulp. Cook for 5–6 minutes. Check seasonings. Remove the mix from the heat and stir in the fresh coriander and leave it to cool.

Fill the tomatoes with the bean mix and place in an oven-proof dish. Bake 15–20 minutes and serve with main course.

4 large beef tomatoes
1 tbsp sunflower oil
225 g onion, chopped
1 garlic clove, crushed
1 pepper, diced
½ tsp each ground cumin and coriander
450 g cooked kidney beans
2 tbsp flour, mixed in a paste with a little water
1 tsp balsamic vinegar
1 bay leaf
4 tbsp fresh chopped coriander
1 pinch each sea salt and pepper

BRING the water to the boil and pour in maize meal. Cook, stirring frequently until it forms a porridge. At this stage, add mashed pumpkin, maple syrup and salt. Combine well and add extra pumpkin water as necessary.

Just before serving, add roasted peanuts and spring onions.

Maize and Pumpkin Meal:
600 ml water
225 g maize or corn meal
325 g cooked, mashed pumpkin (retain cooking water)
½ tsp maple syrup
2 tbsp roasted peanuts
4 tbsp chopped spring onions
1 pinch each sea salt and pepper

— CORIANDER AND BROAD BEAN MOUSSE WITH CORN PASTA —

2 tbsp olive oil
1 tbsp black sesame seeds
175 g diced onions
2 garlic cloves, crushed
sea salt and pepper
1 tsp cumin powder
675 g broad beans, cooked and skinned
2 tbsp chopped fresh coriander
1 tsp lemon juice
1 tbsp agar agar, dissolved in 4 tbsp water

OIL four individual ramekin dishes lightly and line the bottom with greaseproof paper discs. Sprinkle some sesame seeds on the bottom of each dish.

Heat the oil in a pan and sauté onions for 5 minutes. Add garlic, salt, pepper and cumin powder and cook over a low heat for 2–3 minutes. Remove from heat.

When cool, put the onion mix in a food processor together with the broad beans, coriander and lemon juice and process until well puréed. Transfer the bean mix to a bowl and check seasonings.

Gently heat the dissolved agar agar mix, taking care not to boil it. Pour the agar agar into the bean mix, stirring until it is well mixed in. Spoon this mix into the ramekins, cover and refrigerate overnight.

Serve by turning out the ramekins onto individual plates over three slices of tomatoes, if you wish. Remove the greaseproof paper and spoon over the sauce (recipe below).

Making the paprika sauce:
2 tbsp olive oil
1 tsp cumin seeds
1 shallot, finely chopped
1 garlic clove, crushed
1 red pepper, chopped
1 tomato, seeded and chopped
4 tbsp white wine
½ tsp paprika
1 tsp tomato purée
170 ml vegetable stock
1 tbsp chopped fresh parsley
4 tbsp soy cream (optional)

HEAT the oil and sauté the cumin seeds for 2 minutes, add shallot, garlic and red pepper. Sweat until softened. Add chopped tomato, salt, wine and paprika and cook for 3–4 minutes, increasing the heat and reducing the wine. Add tomato purée and vegetable stock. Bring to the boil, lower heat and simmer for 5–10 minutes.

Cool the sauce before blending in a food processor together with chopped parsley. You can pass the sauce through a sieve or otherwise, whilst still warm, you can add soy cream to give it a creamy texture. Spoon it around the green bean mould.

COMBINE the pasta and vegetables. Combine the pasta dressing ingredients well and pour over the pasta. Toss and stir thoroughly. Serve with the rest of menu.

For the corn pasta:
450 g corn pasta, cooked as per packet instructions and drained
100 g spring onions, slivered
4 tbsp chopped sun-dried tomatoes
100 g cubed carrot
225 g watercress, washed and dried

For the pasta dressing:
4 tbsp extra-virgin olive oil
2 garlic cloves, crushed
4 tbsp pine nuts, toasted
4 tbsp chopped fresh parsley
1 tsp lemon juice
1 tbsp tomato purée
2 tbsp water

— BEETROOT MOUSSE WITH RICE SALAD —

PUT the beetroots and soy milk or water in a large pan over a medium heat. Bring to the boil, reduce heat and simmer until tender (45 minutes to 1 hour).

Put the cooked beetroot mix together with the liquid, walnuts and soy sauce into a blender and blend until smooth. Transfer this mix to a bowl.

Heat the agar agar and water mix over a low heat for about 3–4 minutes until well dissolved but not boiling. Combine agar-agar with beetroot mix and pour into individual serving dishes to set. Chill overnight or for a couple of hours. Serve with lemon slices and a ring of rice salad (recipe below).

3–4 beetroots, washed, peeled and diced
150 ml plain soy milk/water
4 tbsp chopped walnuts
2 tbsp soy sauce
2½ tbsp agar agar, dissolved in 150 ml water
2 lemon slices

Making the rice salad:
450 g cooked rice
4 spring onions, chopped
100 g cooked mung beans
100 g carrot, steamed and finely
chopped
100 g fresh peas, steamed
100 g cherry tomatoes, cut in
halves
3 tbsp sunflower oil
sea salt and pepper

For the dressing:
100 g fresh corn kernels, roasted
100 g cashews, roasted
1 tsp grated fresh root ginger
6 tbsp sunflower oil
1 garlic clove, chopped
2 tbsp tamari sauce
1 tbsp coriander
juice of ½ lemon
4 tbsp water

To the cooked cooled rice, add all vegetables and sunflower oil. Season well. Chill for at least 1 hour.

Put all the dressing ingredients in a blender and process until smooth. Add more water if required. Add to cooked rice and vegetables. Serve at room temperature with accompaniments.

— BAKED BROCCOLI AND CAULIFLOWER WITH TOFU SAUCE AND BUTTER BEANS IN ONION GRAVY —

450 g broccoli florets
100 g small cauliflower florets
100 g tofu
2 tbsp sunflower oil
2 tbsp soy sauce
1 tsp mustard powder
4 tbsp sunflower seeds

HEAT some water in a large saucepan, plunge cauliflower florets for 5–8 minutes, just enough time so they are tender, not mushy. Run them immediately under cold water.

Next par-boil broccoli florets in boiling water for 3–4 minutes and plunge them in a pan of cold water. Drain well.

Combine tofu, six tablespoons of cooking water from the cauliflower or broccoli, oil, soy sauce and mustard in a blender. Combine until creamy.

Arrange broccoli and cauliflower in a heat-proof dish, pour over the tofu sauce, sprinkle with sunflower seeds and place under a medium grill until browned.

HEAT the oil in a pan, stir in onion and cook until slightly brown. Add mushrooms, salt and rosemary. Sauté for 6–8 minutes.

Stir in the flour and cook, stirring until it turns brown. Remove pan from the heat and stir in miso and stock. Mix well. Return to heat, bring to the boil and simmer. Add cooked beans and simmer for another 8–10 minutes. Serve with chopped parsley and seasonings.

For the butter beans in onion gravy:
4 tbsp olive oil
225 g finely chopped red onion
450 g halved mushrooms
¼ tsp dried rosemary
1 tbsp wholemeal flour
2 tbsp white miso
375 ml stock
450 g cooked butter beans
sea salt and pepper
chopped fresh parsley, to garnish

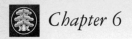 *Chapter 6*

LATE SUMMER

ALTHOUGH *not strictly recognised as a season, late summer is the time when the* yang *energy slowly turns into* yin *quality that will characterise the autumn and winter months. This is the point of transition between the radiance and expansion of summer and the cooler, more mysterious end of summer which announces the autumn to come. There is a timeless, dreamlike, magical quality about this time of year. Now we return from our holidays and prepare for the cooler seasons ahead. It is the time for solitary or intimate walks in forests, wearing an extra layer of clothing. In certain parts of Europe and the United States, late summer is a time of storms, dangerous sea tides and rains. This is the time for contemplation, so allow change to come slowly to your life, relationships and activities.*

To attune to late summer the diet should contain more cooked foods, more protein, less dairy foods and the right combination of carbohydrates.

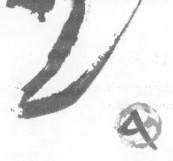

— LATE SUMMER COOKING METHODS —

Boiling, grilling, sautéing, simmering.

— LATE SUMMER FOODS —

Squash, tomatoes, courgettes, carrots, cabbage, peas, chestnuts, corn, sweet potatoes, pumpkin, parsnips.

— LATE SUMMER GRAINS —

Most varieties of legumes.

— LATE SUMMER FRUITS —

Apples, grapes, chestnuts, plums.

— SPECIAL FOODS —

Onions, leeks, ginger, cinnamon, fennel, cooked fruits, barley malt, molasses, rice syrup.

— SUGGESTED BODY THERAPIES —

Loosening and stretching exercises, centring meditations, prana healing, breathing exercises.

— SUGGESTED DIET —

Rice salads, pasta, grain croquettes, buckwheat pancakes, scrambled tofu, tempeh sandwiches.

LUNCH

— GREEN BEAN SALAD —

12 button onions, peeled

3 tbsp extra-virgin olive oil

1 tbsp icing sugar

4 tbsp balsamic vinegar

6 tbsp stock

450 g topped, tailed and sliced French beans

450 g jicama, sliced *

4 tbsp chopped sun-dried tomatoes

sea salt and pepper

lettuce, to serve

BLANCH the button onions in boiling water for 1 minute. Heat the oil in a frying pan, add drained onions and cook until lightly browned. Add sugar and vinegar and allow onions to caramelise. Pour in the stock and cook on a low heat.

Blanch the trimmed beans in boiling water for about 4 minutes. Drain and run them under cold water. Add them to onions, together with sliced jicama and sun-dried tomatoes. Mix well and adjust seasonings. Remove from the heat and serve over a bed of lettuce.

* The jicama is a tuberous vegetable with brown skin and white flesh. It is crisp and crunchy in taste. It can be eaten raw or slightly sautéed. It is very popular in Latin American recipes, but it can be substituted with water chestnuts.

— LUNCHTIME RICE NOODLE SALAD —

BLEND the marinade ingredients well, combine with the tofu and leave in the refrigerator for 2 hours or overnight.

Heat two tablespoons of oil. Add drained tofu and ginger and sauté until tofu is slightly browned. Pour in a little more of marinade (1–2 tsp) and cook for 2 more minutes.

Cook noodles in boiling water as per instructions on the packet. Drain when *al dente*. Add remaining sesame oil, tamari sauce and lemon juice. Toss well.

Mix tofu and vegetables — mangetouts, beansprouts and cucumber — with noodles, adding rest of the marinade ingredients and fresh herbs.

325 g tofu, cut into 1 cm cubes
4 tbsp sesame oil
2 x 150 g packs rice noodles
6 spring onions, chopped
225 g mangetouts, sliced in half diagonally
100 g beansprouts
100 g cucumber thinly sliced and seeded, drained of excess water
2 tbsp tamari sauce
2 tbsp lemon juice
100 g chopped fresh herbs
For the marinade:
4 tbsp cider vinegar
4 tbsp tamari sauce
1 garlic clove, chopped
1 tsp grated root ginger

— TABBOULEH —

IN a large bowl place couscous and pour the boiling water to cover. Let it stand, covered, for 30 minutes or until all the water is absorbed. Stir occasionally.

Uncover and fluff the grain with a fork. Add all the vegetables and herbs. Next add seasonings. Toss and mix well. Serve chilled.

450 g couscous
900 ml boiling water
½ cucumber, peeled, de-seeded and chopped
6 spring onions, sliced
3 tbsp chopped mint
8 cherry tomatoes, halved
100 g currants, soaked in boiling water
225 g green peas, steamed
4 tbsp chopped dried apricots
100 g chopped fresh parsley
1 tsp sea salt
1 tsp cumin powder
6 tbsp lemon juice
4 tbsp olive oil

— WHEATBERRY SALAD —

225 g wheatberries
225 g mung beans
2 celery sticks, finely chopped
2 carrots, diced
100 g chopped fresh parsley
sea salt and pepper
For the dressing:
4 tbsp olive oil
4 tbsp lemon juice
3 garlic cloves, chopped
4 tbsp chopped spring onion
2 tbsp soy sauce
½ tsp mustard
1 tsp cinnamon powder

PUT the wheatberries in a saucepan and cover well with water. Bring to the boil and simmer covered until all the water is absorbed and the grain is tender (about 1 hour). Top it up in-between with water.

Boil the mung beans in a separate pan for about 20 minutes. When the beans and berries are done, remove from heat and drain thoroughly. Mix the vegetables with the cooked grain and beans in a large bowl. Add parsley, salt and pepper. Whisk all the dressing ingredients well and pour over the mixed salad. Toss well and let it stand for some time for the flavours to blend.

— WILD RICE AND QUINOA SALAD —

100 g rinsed wild rice
900 ml water
100 g quinoa
1 tbsp sea salt
pepper
2 tbsp sunflower oil
450 g sliced wild mushrooms
2 garlic cloves, crushed
2 tbsp chopped fresh parsley
4 tbsp toasted pumpkin seeds
100 g chopped red pepper, roasted

PLACE the rice in a pan with 600 ml of water. Bring to the boil and simmer for about 45 minutes to 1 hour until tender. Add more water if needed. Remove from heat and let it stand. In a separate pan bring 300 ml water to the boil with salt. Add the quinoa. Cover and cook on a low heat for 15 minutes.

Heat the oil in a pan and add sliced mushrooms with garlic, salt and parsley and sauté for about 4–5 minutes, stirring continuously. Transfer mushroom mix to a large bowl, add pumpkin seeds and roast peppers. Mix well. Next add cooked grains. Adjust seasonings and serve with tomato and cucumber salad, if you like.

DINNER

STARTERS

— BAKED SPRING ROLLS —

PREHEAT oven to 180°C/350°F/Gas Mark 4. Oil a baking tray. Heat a wok on high temperature. Add sesame oil and lower the heat. Then add ginger, leek and onion and stir-fry for several minutes. Next add carrots and cabbage and stir-fry briefly before adding bean sprouts and spring onions. Add tamari sauce, pepper and rice wine vinegar. Mix well and set aside to cool.

To make spring rolls, fill a large bowl with warm water and dip one of the rice wrappers in the water to soften. Remove from water and drain on a tea towel. Put about two tablespoons of filling on each softened rice wrapper. Fold in each side and roll tightly – they will seal on their own. The rolls should be about 7.5 cm long. Repeat until all filling is used.

Keep the rolls under a moist tea towel until ready to go into the oven. Lightly brush them with olive oil and bake for about 3 minutes on each side. Serve sliced with dipping sauce (recipe follows), lettuce and mint leaves.

COMBINE all ingredients well in a bowl.

1 packet rice paper wrappers
(sold frozen in oriental
supermarkets)
2 tbsp sesame oil
1 tsp grated fresh root ginger
1 leek, cut into very thin slithers
1 white onion, finely sliced
450 g shredded carrots
450 g shredded green cabbage
450 g beansprouts
4 spring onions, chopped
4 tbsp tamari sauce
1 tsp pepper
1 tsp rice wine vinegar

For the sauce:
1 tbsp tamari sauce
2 tbsp cider vinegar
2 garlic cloves, chopped
3 tbsp roasted chopped peanuts
½ tbsp Dijon mustard
2 tsp honey
1 tbsp water
1 tbsp chopped spring onions

— SOY FALAFEL —

2 tbsp sesame oil
225 g chopped onions
675 g firm tofu, mashed
225 g breadcrumbs
4 tbsp chopped fresh parsley
2 tbsp tamari sauce
4 garlic cloves, chopped
1 tbsp each ground cumin and
coriander
4 tbsp tahini
4 tbsp lemon juice
sea salt and pepper

PREHEAT oven to 180°C/350°F/Gas Mark 4 and oil a baking sheet. Fry the onions on a medium heat until soft. Mix all remaining ingredients together and form into 2.5 cm balls.

Bake these falafels in a preheated oven, turning them often so that they are evenly browned on all sides. Remove when golden and serve with hoummus and salad.

— YAM AND WALNUT SALAD —

½ tsp salt
½ tsp sugar
675 g diced sweet potato (also
known as yams)
4 tbsp roasted crushed walnuts
4 tbsp juniper berries, soaked in
water
4 tbsp currants
4 tbsp maple syrup
4 tbsp water
1 tsp cayenne pepper
2 tbsp fruit juice
2 tbsp lemon juice
chopped fresh coriander

BRING a large pan of water to the boil, add salt and sugar and blanch the sweet potatoes for 8–10 minutes. Drain and run them under cold running water. Transfer to a salad bowl. Add walnuts, berries and currants to the bowl with the sweet potatoes.

Heat maple syrup, water and cayenne pepper over a medium heat until the liquid is reduced by half. Cool briefly. Add this to the bowl with the yams and the walnuts and pour fruit and lemon juices over the salad. Add freshly chopped coriander and adjust seasonings. Toss well and serve.

— POTATO CAKES WITH SPINACH SAUCE —

HEAT oil in a frying pan and sauté onion or leeks until soft.

Mash the potatoes, add chopped olives, tomatoes, capers, half the breadcrumbs and cooked leeks (or onions). Season with herbs, salt and pepper. Mix well.

Shape into 1 cm thick patties of desired size. Dip them in egg white and sprinkle with the remaining breadcrumbs. Shallow fry or grill them evenly on both sides for 5 minutes on each side.

1 tbsp sunflower oil
225 g diced red onion (or leeks)
450 g potatoes, boiled
30 olives, pitted and chopped
4 tbsp chopped sun-dried
tomatoes
4 tbsp capers, drained
225 g fresh breadcrumbs
4 tbsp fresh parsley
2 egg whites, beaten
sea salt and pepper

STEAM the spinach briefly. Put it in a food processor together with soy milk, nutmeg and seasoning. Blend well. Warm this sauce and spoon onto warm plates. Place potato cakes on top.

For the spinach sauce:
900 g chopped spinach
4 tbsp soy milk
½ tsp nutmeg
sea salt and pepper

— AUBERGINE CROSTINI —

RUB the garlic clove over each slice of baguette and brush lightly with olive oil. Toast on both sides. Coat aubergine slices well with oil and grill on both sides until brown.

On each toasted baguette place a slice of grilled aubergine, top it evenly with a spoonful of sun-dried tomato purée. Sprinkle with salt, pepper and basil leaves. Return to grill for 2 minutes. Serve warm with a drizzle of olive oil and green salad.

1 small baguette, sliced into thin
oval slices
1 garlic clove
4 tbsp olive oil
1 small aubergine, cut into shape
for bread slices
4 tbsp puréed sun-dried tomatoes
2 tbsp chopped fresh basil

— MARROWS FILLED WITH RICE IN A TOMATO, CAPER AND BLACK OLIVE SAUCE —

1 medium marrow (approx.
1.125kg)
4 tbsp sunflower oil
225 g chopped onions
1 garlic clove, chopped
1 celery stick, chopped
225 g sliced mushrooms
2 tsp mild curry powder
2 small carrots, diced and
steamed
4 tbsp green peas, steamed
325 g cooked brown rice
4 tbsp chopped fresh parsley
2 tbsp chopped hazelnuts
1 pinch each sea salt and pepper

PREHEAT oven to 180°C/350°F/Gas Mark 4. Cut the marrow in half lengthways and scoop out the pith and seeds. Sprinkle with salt and leave upside down to drain for 15–20 minutes. Drain and steam them for 15 minutes and then wipe dry.

While the marrow is draining and steaming, prepare the filling. Heat a wok, add half the oil and sauté onions and garlic until soft. Add celery and mushrooms and stir-fry adding the curry powder and salt.

When vegetables are soft, add carrots and peas. Mix well. Stir in rice, parsley and nuts and season well. Remove from the heat. Press this filling into one half of the marrow. Top it with the other half. Soaked toothpicks can be used to keep the marrow together.

Brush the marrow with oil and place in a roasting tin. Bake for 30–40 minutes and serve with the sauce (recipe below).

For the sauce:
4 tbsp sunflower oil
225 g chopped red onion
2 garlic cloves, chopped
½ tsp dried oregano
6 medium tomatoes, peeled,
seeded and chopped
4 tbsp pitted black olives
2 tbsp capers
½ red chilli, seeded and
chopped (optional)
black pepper

HEAT the oil in a pan. Add onions, garlic, salt and oregano. Cook for 3–4 minutes, stirring. Add tomatoes and cook for an additional 3 minutes. Add olives, capers and chilli (optional) and simmer for 15–20 minutes until the sauce is thick (or pour over the marrow and bake). Add black pepper.

— VEGETABLE PANZEROTTI WITH GLAZED BEETROOT —

COOK the spinach with a little oil in a frying pan for 5–6 minutes. Squeeze out all excess water. Chop the cooked spinach and place in a bowl. Add garlic, capers, olives, nuts and raisins. Adjust seasonings.

On a clean work surface, roll out the pizza dough until very thin. Using a biscuit cutter, cut the dough into circles. Leaving the borders of the dough clean, place a tablespoon of spinach filling in the middle. Brush the beaten egg along the border of each circle. Fold in half and seal well. Use a fork to seal it.

Heat some oil in a pan and deep fry the panzerotti until golden brown. Alternatively bake the panzerotti in a pre-heated oven (180°C/350°F/Gas Mark 4) for 15–20 minutes.

450 g spinach, washed and trimmed
150 ml sunflower oil
2 garlic cloves, crushed
1 tbsp capers
4 tbsp pitted chopped olives
2 tbsp crushed roasted walnuts
1 tbsp raisins, soaked in water and chopped
Wholewheat pizza dough (see page 60)
1 egg, beaten
sea salt and pepper

PREHEAT oven to 180°C/350°F/Gas Mark 4. Place coarsely grated beetroot in an oven-proof dish. Add red wine, vinegar, sugar, oil and seasonings. Cover with a lid or tin foil. Bake in preheated oven for 20–30 minutes, stirring occasionally. Before serving, add orange zest.

For the glazed beetroot:
675 g peeled and grated raw beetroot
4 tbsp red wine
2 tbsp rice vinegar
1 tbsp sugar
2 tbsp sunflower oil
2 tbsp raisins or cranberries, soaked in water
orange rind
sea salt and pepper

— TERIYAKI TOFU WITH MARINATED
GRILLED VEGETABLES —

*2 blocks firm or smoked tofu,
drained and cut into chunks*

COOK the tofu under a grill under browned on all sides.

For the Teriyaki marinade:
300 ml tamari sauce
150 ml white wine
4 tbsp honey
1 tbsp grated root ginger
6 garlic cloves, chopped
1 tsp mustard powder
100 g grated onions
pepper

COMBINE all ingredients for marinade and bring them to the boil. Simmer for 5–8 minutes. Pour the hot marinade over tofu cubes. Toss well and let it sit overnight in the refrigerator.

For the grilled vegetables:
*10 mushrooms, cut in half and
wiped clean*
1 red pepper, cut into wedges
*10 button onions, peeled and
parboiled*
*225 g cubed winter squash,
boiled for 5 minutes*
8 cherry tomatoes
1 spring onion, chopped
2 tbsp sunflower oil
*1 tbsp each chopped fresh parsley
and thyme*
1 tbsp Dijon mustard
1 tbsp sherry vinegar

POUR the minimum amount of oil over the mushrooms, pepper, onions, winter squash and tomatoes. Grill all the vegetables. Make the dressing by blending the spring onion, oil, herbs, mustard and sherry vinegar. Dress the grilled vegetables, tossing well so that they are well coated.

— PAELLA WITH SUMMER SALAD —

HEAT oil in a large pan and fry onions and garlic for a few minutes. Add rice, cashew nuts, paprika and turmeric. Mix well and cook, stirring, for a few minutes. Add basil and remaining vegetables and mix well.

Pour puréed tomato and vegetable stock into pan. Simmer for 35–40 minutes or until the vegetables and rice are tender and water has evaporated.

Serve warm with olives, lemon wedges, hard-boiled egg and parsley.

2 tbsp olive oil
225 g chopped onions
2 garlic cloves, crushed
100 g long grain brown rice
100 g chopped cashew nuts
½ tsp paprika
½ tsp turmeric
chopped fresh basil
1 red and 1 green pepper, cut into strips
4 celery sticks, diced
2 courgettes, diced
1 large carrot, diced
100 g green peas
4–6 tomatoes, skinned, de-seeded and puréed
600 ml vegetable stock (see page 58)
1 tbsp whole green olives
lemon wedges
hard-boiled egg, sliced
chopped fresh parsley
sea salt and pepper

COMBINE the lettuce, celery, cucumber, avocado, tomatoes and the spring onions and toss thoroughly with the French Dressing.

For the Summer Salad:
1 small head lettuce, washed, dried and torn into bite-size pieces
3 celery sticks, chopped
¼ cucumber, diced
1 avocado, cut into chunks
2 tomatoes, sliced
1 bunch spring onions, sliced
French Dressing (see page 48)

— SOBA NOODLES WITH SPINACH ROLLS AND SESAME SAUCE —

400 g soba noodles

1 litre Japanese Stock (see page 59)

5 tbsp sesame oil

1 onion, sliced

2 carrots, cut into matchsticks

450 g shredded white cabbage

6–8 shiitake mushrooms

½ tsp Japanese five-spice powder

4 tbsp chopped spring onions

100 g grated radish or daikon

sea salt and pepper

COOK noodles in a large pan. Follow instructions on the packet and cook until *al dente* – about 6–7 minutes. Drain in a colander.

Heat three tablespoons of oil in a large frying pan, add noodles and with the help of tongs, stir-fry for 2–3 minutes. Add salt and pepper. Keep warm but do not overcook.

Heat the remaining oil in a frying pan and stir-fry onion, carrots, cabbage and mushrooms together with Japanese five-spice powder. Stir-fry 3–4 minutes. Add noodles and toss the mix well over the heat. Transfer to a serving dish. Sprinkle with spring onion and grated daikon. Serve with sesame sauce on the side (see following recipe).

For the sesame sauce:

5 tbsp white sesame seeds

170 ml dashi

6 tbsp tamari sauce

2 tbsp mirin

1 tbsp sugar

1–2 tbsp sake

IN a heavy frying pan, roast the white sesame seeds until golden brown. Keep moving the pan to avoid burning. Transfer these to a grinding bowl and using a pestle, grind them until flaky.

Add remaining ingredients and whisk well.

BRING some salted water to the boil. Add spinach and simmer for 2 minutes. Plunge into cold water and squeeze out excess water. In the same boiling water, add the cabbage leaves and cook for 2–3 minutes until just tender. Plunge into cold water to get a bright green colour. Pat dry.

Lay cabbage leaves on a work surface. Sprinkle with gomasio, then spread spinach over each leaf. Tightly roll each cabbage leaf, starting from stalk end. Squeeze all excess water. Use a Japanese sushi rolling mat to make the job easier. With a sharp knife, cut each roll into four pieces. Sprinkle with gomasio.

For the spinach rolls:
300 g fresh spinach, washed
4 large Chinese cabbage leaves
4 tbsp gomasio (a condiment made from roasted sesame seeds and sea salt available from health food stores)
sea salt

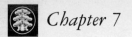

Chapter 7

AUTUMN

THE *23 September on the equinox, announces the harvesting season and the beginning of the* yin *energy which will grow progressively stronger over the next six months. Temperatures drop and the colours of nature change dramatically, from dark greens to all hues of orange, red and brown – nature is magnificent before its winter death. This is a time to stock your pantry with herbs, grains and legumes for the cold months ahead, to store up on fuel, prepare your wardrobe for the rainy season and winter and to repair your house against any leaks and draughts.*

Autumn activities are mostly indoors, except for walks in the forests and the last hours spent in the garden protecting your plants for the cold to come. It is now that we read, write letters and plan with family and friends in front of blazing fires.

Autumn is the season for fragrant kitchen smells – mulled wine, baking and roasting chestnuts on open fires. In order to focus mentally and stimulate activity of the body, eat stews and lightly baked foods.

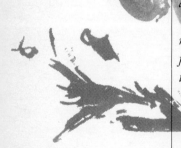

— AUTUMN COOKING METHODS —

Simmer, baking, sautéing – less water and more heat.

— AUTUMN FOODS —

Onions, squash, turnips, mushrooms, spinach, cauliflower.

— AUTUMN GRAINS —

Rice, rye, bulgar, cracked wheat.

— AUTUMN FRUITS —

Apples, limes, pears, chestnuts, hazelnuts, persimmons, pine nuts, almonds, sesame seeds.

— SPECIAL FOODS —

Soybean products – tofu, tempeh and soy milk – to combat dryness; also spinach, barley, millet, pears, sea vegetables, almonds, pine nuts, barley malt and rice syrup.

— AUTUMN HERBS —

Rosemary, ginger, burdock, comfrey.

— SUGGESTED BODY THERAPIES —

Dancing, yoga, breathing exercises, stretching, singing, humming, sitting meditations.

Flavoured foods, sauerkraut, umeboshi (see page 175), rose-hip tea, grilled sandwiches, couscous, millet pilaff, aduki beans.

LUNCH

— LENTIL PÂTÉ SANDWICHES —

325 g diced onions
½ tsp cumin seeds
2 tbsp olive oil
325 g lentils
150 ml water
1 tsp salt
2 tsp tamari sauce
1 tbsp garlic powder
1 tsp celery seeds
1 tsp mixed dried herbs
soy garlic mayonnaise (see page 43)
1 lettuce, shredded
1 tomato, sliced
red onion rings

IN a large saucepan sauté onion and cumin seeds in hot oil.

Grind the lentils to a fine consistency with a blender or a pestle and mortar. Add them to the pan with water and add rest of the seasonings – tamari sauce, garlic powder, celery seeds and mixed herbs. Bring to the boil and simmer covered for 1 hour.

Transfer the contents to a loaf pan and chill overnight or few hours until firm.

To serve, invert the loaf pan onto a serving platter and slice. Grill to brown the top.

Assemble the sandwich by spreading soy mayonnaise on each slice. Layer the bread slices with shredded lettuce and tomato. Top with grilled lentil pâté. Top with onion rings. Cover with another slice of bread. Cut in half and serve with a dressed lettuce salad.

— WARM WHOLEWHEAT PITTA WITH BEANS —

HEAT oil over a low heat. Sweat onions, turnips and garlic for 10 minutes. Stir in the cooked beans together with horseradish. Stir and mix well. Add parsley and pickled onions before adding the stock and seasoning. Cover and cook for 20 minutes. Mash the mix with the back of a wooden spoon.

Warm the pitta. Slit it open and spread with the bean mix. Top it with crunchy salad and serve.

2 tbsp sunflower oil
225 g diced onions
225 g scrubbed and diced white turnips
1 garlic clove, chopped
450 g soaked and cooked black-eyed beans
1 tbsp grated horseradish sauce
2 tbsp chopped fresh parsley
4 pickling onions, chopped
450 ml vegetable stock (see page 58)
2 pitta breads
lettuce
sea salt and pepper

— WARM SPICY CABBAGE ROLLS —

HEAT oil in a heavy skillet. Add mustard and cumin seeds. When they start to pop, add turmeric, cabbage and other seasonings. Stir-fry for 8–10 minutes.

Brush the chapatis or burritos with olive oil and warm them in the oven. Assemble the rolls by rolling the cooked cabbage into warm bread. Sprinkle with fresh coriander.

You can also use hoummus as a spread for added flavour (see page 44).

2 tsp sunflower oil
½ tsp mustard seeds
½ tsp cumin seeds
½ tsp turmeric
1 medium cabbage, shredded
1 tsp salt
2 tsp ground coriander
1 tbsp lemon juice
4–6 flat bread-like chapatis or burritos (available in most supermarkets or delicatessens)
olive oil
chopped fresh coriander

— HOT POTATO SALAD —

20 small new potatoes, scrubbed
6 tbsp sunflower oil
2 garlic cloves, crushed
1 tbsp lemon juice
½ tsp wholegrain mustard
1 tbsp balsamic vinegar
½ tsp honey
2 tbsp chopped fresh parsley
2 tbsp chopped olives
6 spring onions, sliced

BOIL or steam baby potatoes until soft, but not mushy.

Whisk rest of the ingredients in a salad bowl and add the warm potatoes when cooked. Toss well. Stand for 30 minutes or more. Serve at room temperature.

— MEDITERRANEAN TOFU ON TOAST —

1 block firm tofu, cubed
1 tsp dried rosemary
4 tbsp olive oil
1 small red onion, sliced
2 garlic cloves, chopped
1 tsp each salt and pepper
1 red and 1 yellow pepper, seeded
and thinly sliced
1 tbsp capers
1 tbsp chopped fresh basil
4 slices crusty herb bread

TOSS tofu and rosemary together with half the oil and grill the dressed tofu evenly on all sides until slightly brown.

Heat rest of the oil and sauté onion, garlic and salt until transparent. Add pepper to the onion mix and cook on low heat for about 8 minutes, stirring often. Towards the end of cooking, add capers, basil and season.

Toast the herb bread lightly. Brush with olive oil. Arrange tofu pieces on the bread and top with pepper and onion mix and fresh basil. Serve covered with another slice of bread.

DINNER

STARTERS

— CABBAGE AND WHITE BEAN SOUP —

HEAT three tablespoons of olive oil in a large saucepan and sauté onions, garlic, carrot, celery and parsley for 4–5 minutes. Add tomato. Stir well and remove from heat within 5 minutes. Purée half the beans and mix with cooked vegetables.

In a large pan heat remaining olive oil. When hot, add caraway seeds, shaking the pan to make sure not to burn the seeds. Add shredded cabbage and quickly stir-fry for 3–4 minutes. Stir in the puréed bean mixture. Cook for 2 minutes.

Add vegetable stock together with 1 litre of the cooking liquid from the beans to the pan with cabbage. Bring to the boil and simmer covered for 20–25 minutes, stirring occasionally. When the cabbage is cooked stir in the remaining beans. Adjust seasonings.

Add corn meal to the soup in a thin stream, stirring constantly to avoid lumps. Simmer for 10–15 minutes. Serve with additional olive oil.

4 tbsp olive oil

225 g chopped onions

3 garlic cloves, chopped

1 carrot, chopped

2 celery sticks, chopped

4 tbsp chopped fresh parsley

4 tbsp peeled and seeded tomato

450 g white beans, soaked overnight and cooked 30 minutes in pressure cooker (reserve the liquid)

4 tbsp caraway seeds

450 g cabbage, shredded

600 ml vegetable stock (see page 58)

4 tbsp corn meal

— MUSHROOMS WITH SWISS CHARD AND ALMONDS —

8 large open mushrooms
2 tbsp olive oil
1 yellow onion, finely chopped
2 garlic cloves, chopped
900 g chopped Swiss chard, washed and drained
4 tbsp finely chopped almonds
1 tbsp lemon juice
4 tbsp pesto
4 tbsp breadcrumbs
2 tbsp chopped fresh parsley

PREHEAT oven to 180°C/350°F/Gas Mark 4. Wipe the mushrooms clean and remove the stalks and save. Lay the caps on an oiled baking tray. Chop the mushroom stalks finely. Heat oil in a wide skillet and add onion and cook on a medium heat until soft. Add garlic and the mushroom stalks and stir well.

Next, add chard leaves. Mix all ingredients well with a pair of tongs. Cook for 7–8 minutes. Dry-roast the chopped almonds and add to the chard. Mix well.

Take the chard off the heat, add the lemon juice and pesto and process in a food processor. Place the mixture in a bowl. Blend the breadcrumbs with the chard mix and spoon it carefully into mushroom caps. Sprinkle with parsley. Bake for 15–18 minutes until the mushrooms are soft and juicy and the top is crispy. Serve warm with garlic bread.

— LEEKS AU GRATIN —

300 ml vegetable stock (see page 58)
10 baby leeks, trimmed and cut in half lengthways and washed
4 tbsp olive oil
2 tbsp breadcrumbs

For the sauce:
2 tbsp chopped shallots
1 tbsp chopped fresh parsley
2 tbsp chopped red pepper
1 tsp English mustard
4 tbsp wine vinegar
4 tbsp olive oil
sea salt and pepper

BRING the vegetable stock to the boil and blanch the leeks for 2–3 minutes. Drain well.

Heat oil in a large pan and cook leeks over a medium heat, stirring occasionally. Cook for 4 minutes. Turn the leeks into a flameproof dish.

Whisk all sauce ingredients and pour over the leeks. Sprinkle with breadcrumbs.

Grill the dish just before serving under a low grill for 2–3 minutes until lightly browned.

Serve warm with fresh seasonal herbs and wholewheat bread.

— CAULIFLOWER AND COCONUT SOUP —

IN a large pan, combine vegetable stock and coconut milk with lemon grass, ginger, garlic, peppercorns, cauliflower, spring onions, soy, sugar and chilli (if wished). Simmer covered for 20 minutes or until cauliflower is soft. Remove from heat, stir in lime juice and serve sprinkled with coriander and chopped spring onions.

600 ml vegetable stock (see page 58)

750 ml coconut milk

2 tbsp chopped dried lemon grass or 2 stalks chopped lime leaves

2 tbsp chopped root ginger

2 garlic cloves, sliced

2 peppercorns, crushed

1 small cauliflower, cut into florets

4 spring onions, chopped

2 tbsp soy sauce

1 tsp sugar

1 red chilli, seeded and chopped (optional)

1 tbsp lime juice

chopped coriander

— DAIKON CAKES IN ORIENTAL SAUCE —

PURÉE the daikon in a food processor. Mix the daikon with the rice and wheat flours. Use water to knead the dough. Transfer the dough into a shallow 20 cm tin and steam over boiling water for 30–35 minutes. To check for readiness, insert a toothpick and see if it comes out clean. When done, remove from the heat and cool. Cut cooked cake into small rectangles.

Heat half the oil in a skillet, add the daikon cake pieces. Fry them until brown. Remove from the pan to a kitchen towel to drain excess oil.

Add rest of the oil and heat. Add garlic, ginger, soy sauce and beansprouts. Toss well and add fried daikon cakes and cook quickly for 1 or 2 minutes. Mix well.

Serve with chopped spring onions if you wish.

1 large daikon, peeled and cut into small cubes

325 g rice flour

2 tbsp wholewheat flour

2 tbsp water

For the oriental sauce:

3 tbsp sesame oil

2 garlic cloves, chopped

2 tbsp finely slivered ginger

4 tbsp soy sauce

4 tbsp beansprouts

4 spring onions, chopped

— FENNEL RISOTTO WITH MUSHROOM AND WATERCRESS BAKE —

6 tbsp olive oil
4 tbsp chopped onion
4 tbsp chopped celery
900 g chopped fennel
550 g Italian arborio rice
150 ml dry white wine
1.5 litres vegetable stock (see page 58)
4 tbsp chopped fresh parsley
1 tbsp lemon juice
sea salt and pepper

HEAT half the oil and sauté onion and celery over a high heat for 3 minutes, stirring often.

Add fennel. Reduce heat and cook for 5 minutes. When fennel begins to brown, lower the heat. Add the rice with the wine and stir until wine is absorbed. Continue by adding the stock gradually, stirring until rice is fully cooked *al dente* – approximately 20 minutes. Do not allow the rice to stick to the pan. Remove from heat and sprinkle with parsley and lemon juice. Serve warm.

For the Mushroom and Watercress Bake:
4 tbsp olive oil
450 g mushrooms, wiped and cut in half
1 tbsp lemon juice
1 tbsp wholemeal flour
1 tsp mustard powder
300 ml soy milk
2 bunches watercress, washed and drained
1 tbsp chopped fresh parsley
sea salt and pepper

PREHEAT oven to 200°C/400°F/Gas Mark 6. Heat half the oil in a frying pan and fry mushrooms for 2 minutes. Pour in lemon juice, let it bubble and get absorbed. Remove mushrooms from heat and with a slotted spoon transfer them to an oven-proof dish. Heat remaining oil, add flour and mustard powder and cook, stirring continuously, for 3–4 minutes. Remove from heat and stir in milk. Stir to avoid lumps. Put it back on the heat and simmer for 4 minutes. Now, fold in watercress and allow it to wilt – about 2 minutes.

Pour the watercress sauce over the mushrooms and place in a hot oven for 20 minutes. Grill the bake for last 5 minutes. Sprinkle salt, pepper and parsley over the top.

— HERBED MILLET PILAFF WITH AVIYAL —

HEAT oil in a heavy-bottomed pan. When hot, add cumin seeds. Lightly fry them and add onion, garlic, ginger and coriander powder. Stir well and add celery and carrot to the onion mix, frying for 6–8 minutes until onions are soft.

Stir in millet together with vegetable stock and salt. Bring to the boil, cover and simmer on a low heat for 30–40 minutes. Extra stock may be needed before millet cooks. When ready, fluff the cooked millet with a fork , stir in remaining ingredients and serve with spicy aviyal (as follows).

For the herbed millet:
2 tbsp olive oil
1 tsp cumin seeds
1 large onion, chopped
2 garlic cloves, chopped
1 tsp grated root ginger
½ tsp ground coriander
2 celery sticks, chopped
1 carrot, grated
225 g dried millet
900 ml vegetable stock (see page 58)
½ tsp sea salt
2 tbsp chopped fresh coriander
chopped fresh parsley
pine nuts
currants

BLEND coconut and water in a blender until smooth. Heat oil in a heavy-based skillet. Add onion, ginger and garlic. Sauté until lightly browned. Add coriander, turmeric, garam masala powder and salt. Mix well and keep cooking for 2–3 minutes.

Next add various chopped vegetables. Mix all the ingredients well for another 2–3 minutes. Stir often, so all vegetables cook evenly. Add coconut and water, purée and bring to the boil. Cover and simmer for 8 minutes. Uncover and add chilli. Serve with the herbed millet.

For the Aviyal:
225 g shredded coconut
300 ml water
1 tbsp olive oil
225 g sliced onions
2 tsp chopped fresh ginger
3 garlic cloves, chopped
2 tsp ground coriander
2 tsp turmeric
1 tbsp garam masala powder (optional)
2 green beans, cut in half lengthways
2 carrots, sliced
225 g diced squash
450 g broccoli florets
1 chilli, seeded and chopped

— KASHI AND SPINACH PASTA WITH STEAMED BEETROOT —

450 g roasted buckwheat kernels
(kashi)

1 bay leaf

1 litre winter vegetable stock (or
stock cube)

½ packet soba noodles

2 tbsp olive oil

225 g sliced onions

450 g halved mushrooms

2 garlic cloves, chopped

1 tbsp wholewheat flour

chopped fresh herbs: thyme,
rosemary, sage, nutmeg

900 g chopped spinach, washed
and well drained

300 ml vegetable stock

nori flakes

HEAT a heavy-bottomed pan and briefly pan-roast the buckwheat, stirring constantly. Add bay leaf and winter stock. Cover and bring to the boil. Reduce heat and simmer for 20 minutes or until kashi is soft. Stir once or twice while cooking.

Prepare the noodles as per the instructions on the packet in a pan of salted boiling water. Heat oil in a pan and sauté onions, add mushrooms, garlic and herbs. Stir well for 2 minutes. Add flour to mushrooms and sauté, stirring until the flour is lightly browned.

By handfuls, add spinach until it wilts. Sprinkle nutmeg over the top and cook on a low heat. Add vegetable stock and bring to the boil. Whisk while gravy reduces in volume.

Combine soba and kashi in a serving dish and ladle over the warm sauce. Toss well with tongs.

Serve with nori flakes.

STEAM the beetroot slices over a pan of boiling water for 25–30 minutes or until tender. Drain well. Whisk together rest of the ingredients.

Arrange beetroot on a serving dish and pour over the dressing. Serve warm.

For the steamed beetroot:
2–3 raw beetroots, washed and sliced
2 tbsp olive oil
2 tbsp lemon juice
1 tsp ground ginger
2 tsp chopped fresh parsley
2 tsp walnuts
1 tsp balsamic vinegar
sea salt and pepper

— CHICKPEA AND POTATO BAKE WITH ARUGULA AND TOMATO SALAD —

PREHEAT oven to 160°C/325°F/Gas Mark 3. Wrap the whole pearl onions in foil with some olive oil and two sprigs of thyme and start baking them. It takes 45 minutes to 1 hour.

Heat half the oil in a skillet. Add onions, celery and carrots with bay leaf and sauté and brown them lightly — about 6–8 minutes.

Next, add mushrooms and garlic with remaining thyme, salt and pepper. Sauté all ingredients for another 6 minutes or until mushrooms are soft. Pour wine over the vegetables and on a medium heat allow it to evaporate for 5–6 minutes.

In an oven-proof dish, put potatoes and chickpeas and combine them with cooked vegetables. Cover with foil and warm them in a preheated oven for 20–25 minutes. Remove and brown lightly under the grill. When done, remove from the heat. Sprinkle with olives, the baked onions and slices of lemon over the top. Serve with the light salad below.

450 g peeled whole pearl onions
4 tbsp olive oil
3 sprigs of thyme
100 g each coarsely diced carrots, celery and onion
1 bay leaf
450 g mushrooms, halved
1 tbsp chopped garlic
150 ml white wine
900 g diced potatoes
450 g cooked chickpeas
4 tbsp pitted green olives
1 lemon
sea salt and pepper

For the Arugula and Tomato
Salad:
1 wholewheat focaccia, cut into
cubes
170 ml mustard vinaigrette
675 g chopped arugula leaves,
washed and dried
225 g thinly sliced onions
2 large tomatoes, chopped

IN a salad bowl, toss focaccia bread cubes with half the vinaigrette and set it aside for a few minutes. Just before serving, add all ingredients together and pour over the salad dressing. Toss well.

— FRIED TOFU IN A MEDITERRANEAN SAUCE —

8–10 thick slices tofu, drained
well
6–8 tbsp wholewheat flour, for
dredging
6 tbsp olive oil
2 tsp chopped garlic
4 tbsp chopped sun-dried
tomatoes
2 tbsp capers
10 oil-preserved artichoke
quarters
170 ml wine
4 tsp lemon juice
4 cups chopped spinach, washed
and spun dried
sea salt and pepper

SEASON the tofu slices with salt and pepper. Dredge them in flour and shake off the excess. Heat oil in a large skillet. Add four tablespoons of oil and fry the tofu slices in batches, turning them over once when lightly browned. Keep fried slices warm in a warm oven.

In the same pan, add remaining oil and add garlic, tomatoes, capers, artichokes, wine and lemon juice. Bring to the boil and simmer for 6–8 minutes.

Meanwhile, steam the spinach until bright green. Season lightly with salt and pepper.

To serve, put spinach in the centre of a dinner plate. Lay tofu slices on the top and pour over the sauce evenly on each plate.

Chapter 8

WINTER

....

THE *solstice on December 21, our longest night, marks the beginning of winter. Yin energy is now at its most potent — everything that is inner, mysterious and dark is emphasised. We dress in warm clothing and limit outdoor activities, except for fun-packed games in the snow and long walks in desolate, silent forests. Animals sleep, the world outside is quiet. This is a time for deep meditation, contemplation, reflection before action. It is time to rest and store physical energy — many put on a little weight during these cold months. We keep our houses warm by keeping constant, even temperatures (not sudden heats and colds), we wear warmer clothes and keep our feet warm. This is the time for hot beverages and stews to prevent chills from ailing us. Winter is a very feminine time — understanding, wisdom and inner strength.*

To attune with winter, we eat wholesome grains, increase fat intake and our meals should be cooked.

— WINTER COOKING METHODS —

Cook longer at lower temperatures with less water. Boiling, steaming, baking, light frying.

— WINTER FOODS —

Carrots, turnips, broccoli, potatoes, kale, onions, cabbage, celery.

— WINTER GRAINS —

Kashi, amaranth, buckwheat, millet, rice.

— WINTER FRUITS —

Apples oranges and dried fruits.

— SPECIAL FOODS —

Protein in the form of tofu, goat's cheese, miso and legumes. Also liquorice, chicory and horsetail for bitter taste. Salty foods such as miso, soy sauce, sea vegetables, millet and barley.

— WINTER HERBS —

Marshmallow root, nettle, herbal teas.

— SUGGESTED BODY THERAPIES —

Choose a warm spot to exercise at home or wear extra layers of clothing when coming out of your workout. Yoga, stretching, deep and still meditations, aromatherapy, *reiki,* deep tissue massage and *shiatsu.*

— SUGGESTED DIET —

Soups, bakes, soba noodles, lentil nut loaf, fried rice, miso soup every day.

— ONE-POT NOODLES —

1 packet udon noodles
1 litre Japanese stock (see page 59)
1 tsp tamari sauce
1 tsp mirin
8–10 shiitake mushrooms, soaked and chopped with stems removed
1 carrot, cut into matchsticks
6 water chestnuts
225 g pumpkin skins
4 spring onions, sliced
225 g shredded cabbage
2 tbsp sesame oil
2 tbsp mustard

COOK udon as per instructions on the packet. Drain and rinse under cold water. Keep in cold water inside a bowl to prevent the noodles from sticking.

Combine stock, tamari sauce and mirin in a pan and start heating on a medium heat. Put in vegetables one by one with cabbage and spring onions last. Cook for 6–8 minutes. To this stock, add noodles, having drained them from the cold water and simmer until heated through.

Serve with additional soy and mustard sauce.

— MOLLETES MEXICO-STYLE —

1 baguette French bread
2 tbsp olive oil
1 tsp cumin seeds
100 g chopped onions
1½ tsp ground coriander
sea salt and pepper
225 g cooked red or black beans, slightly mashed
2–4 tbsp chopped tomatoes
100 g non-dairy cheese (optional)

HEAT oven to 180°C/350°F/Gas Mark 4. Slice the baguette into four and then slice each piece in half lengthways. Scoop out some bread from each piece to make eight cradles.

Heat oil in a skillet. When hot, add cumin seeds and as soon as they change colour, add onions followed by coriander, salt and pepper. Fry until onions are lightly browned. Add coarsely mashed beans and chopped tomatoes. Cook for 6–8 minutes, stirring often. When beans are ready, fill the hollow in the bread with the mixture, topped with the optional non-dairy cheese. Place bread in the oven until heated through or under a grill until the top browns.

— NUT BURGERS —

PREHEAT oven to 180°C/350°F/Gas Mark 4. Fry onions and garlic in hot oil together with coriander and mustard powder until soft. Stir in the flour and cook stirring for 2–3 minutes.

Pour the water or stock in a stream and bring to the boil. Remove from heat, stir in remaining ingredients, adjust seasonings and let stand until cold.

Shape this mix into round burgers and place on greased baking sheet. Cook in preheated oven for about 25 minutes, turn them over after 15 minutes to cook evenly on all sides. Serve warm or at room temperature with raw salad and a dressing of your choice.

225 g chopped onions

1 garlic clove, crushed

2 tbsp olive oil

1 tsp ground coriander

1 tsp mustard powder

4 tbsp flour

150 ml water or stock

450 g chopped mixed nuts

225 g fresh breadcrumbs

450 g coarsely grated carrots

1 tbsp chopped fresh parsley

1 tbsp lemon juice

— SANDWICHES OF FRIED FENNEL AND SALAD —

BRING a pan of water to the boil. Add fennel bulbs and boil for not more than 3–4 minutes. Drain well. Dredge fennel slices in flour. Shake the excess flour and set aside.

Heat the oil until very hot. Add fennel slices and fry until golden on all sides. Remove and drain on paper towels.

Lightly toast the bread. Brush with olive oil, add the fennel slices and top with the slices of tomato. Grill until tomato slices are charred. Season well and serve.

2 fennel bulbs, trimmed and cut into 2.5 cm thick wedges

4 tbsp wholewheat flour

8 tbsp olive oil

1 tomato, sliced

crusty Italian bread

sea salt and pepper

— AUBERGINE AND HOUMMUS SANDWICHES —

1 large aubergine, sliced
6–8 tbsp olive oil
1 garlic clove, chopped
2 tbsp chopped fresh parsley
1 tbsp chopped fresh basil
1 tbsp lemon juice
balsamic vinegar
4–6 tbsp hoummus
4–6 slices wholewheat bread
sea salt and pepper

PLACE the aubergine in a colander and sprinkle with salt. Let it stand for 30 minutes. Drain well and pat dry.

Heat oil in a large frying pan. Add garlic and aubergine slices and sauté, turning over when one side is browned. Remove cooked slices and place them on paper towels with a slotted spoon to drain excess oil. Season with herbs, salt, pepper, lemon juice and vinegar.

While the aubergine is cooking, lightly toast the bread and spread hoummus thinly on the slices.

To assemble the sandwich, put two slices of aubergine on each slice of bread and top with another slice of bread and serve with a salad and a dressing of your choice.

DINNER

STARTERS

— CARROT AND PARSNIP CAKES WITH SHALLOT AND PLUM SAUCE —

3 carrots, peeled and diced
3 parsnips, peeled and diced
2 tbsp olive oil
chopped fresh parsley
sea salt and pepper
225 g self-raising flour

COOK carrots and parsnips in boiling water until tender. Mash well, add oil, herbs and seasonings. Cool.

On a floured board, work in the vegetable mix and flour. Knead well and let it stand until ready to cook. Roll out the dough and cut into 1 cm thick round cakes and cook under a grill for 3–4 minutes on each side.

HEAT oil and fry shallots and garlic. Remove from heat. Whisk together all ingredients and serve on side with carrot and parsnip cakes.

For the Shallot and Plum Sauce:
1 tbsp olive oil
3 shallots
2 garlic cloves, chopped
4 tbsp plum sauce (available in supermarkets or oriental stores)
2 tbsp water
soy sauce, to flavour
⅛ chilli, chopped

— LENTIL PARCELS WITH A CORIANDER DIPPING SAUCE —

HEAT half the oil and add mustard seeds. Just when they start to pop, add onion and stir well. Fry for 2 minutes.

Next add spinach in small batches with ginger root and nutmeg. Stir well and cook until the spinach has wilted. Stir in red lentils and salt and pepper. Cook briefly for 4–5 minutes. Remove from heat and cool. Place a teaspoon of this mix in the centre of each wonton wrapper. Brush the edges with egg mix and gather up all four ends and press firmly.

4 tbsp olive oil
2 tsp mustard seeds
8 spring onions, chopped
450 g finely chopped spinach
2 tsp grated fresh ginger
½ tsp grated nutmeg
225 g cooked red lentils
10–15 wonton wrappers (sold frozen in oriental supermarkets)
sea salt and pepper
1 egg, lightly beaten

BLEND all ingredients together in a food processor until smooth. Adjust seasonings. Thin it with water or coconut milk to get desired consistency. Place dipping sauce in individual small bowls to go with each set of lentil parcels.

For the Coriander Dipping Sauce:
450 g chopped fresh coriander
4 tbsp lemon juice
4 tbsp grated coconut
2 tbsp grated root ginger
1 tsp honey
1 tsp each sea salt and pepper

— CELERIAC SOUP —

3 tbsp olive oil

5 leeks, with white parts only, sliced

1 fennel, trimmed and sliced

½ tsp fennel seeds

1 tsp celery seeds

2 garlic cloves, crushed

1 tsp salt

2 tbsp chopped fresh parsley

1 litre Winter Vegetable Stock (see page 58)

2 tbsp chopped inner fennel leaves

1 small celery head, trimmed and sliced

HEAT two tablespoons of oil and sauté leeks until they become brighter in colour. Add fennel, fennel seeds, celery seeds and garlic, salt and parsley. Stirring often, let the vegetables cook for 4–5 minutes.

Add 150 ml of stock along with fennel leaves and celery head. Cover and simmer for 20 minutes. Check for water while simmering.

Add stock to simmering vegetables, cover and cook for a further 15 minutes. Blend the soup in a food processor after it has cooled.

If blended soup is too thick, add some more stock. Heat it through and serve with sweet onions (recipe below).

For Sweet Onions:

1 large sweet onion, peeled and finely sliced

1 tbsp olive oil

TOSS onion and oil well and lay them on a baking sheet.

Grill, turning often until just lightly browned — about 12–15 minutes or cook them in oven at 150°C/300°F/Gas Mark 2, again turning often.

— SPLIT PEA SOUP —

HEAT oil in a large pan and sauté onion and garlic. Next add celery, carrots and parsnip with a touch of salt and nutmeg. Stir well. Brown the vegetables very slightly.

Stir in drained split peas followed by stock, add pepper. Bring to the boil, cover and simmer. Cook for 1½ hours or so. If required, add more stock or water to thin the soup.

Purée about ¼ of the soup in a blender, add to the rest of the soup, bring back to the heat and adjust seasonings.

Serve with parsley and coriander, generously sprinkled.

2 tbsp olive oil

225 g diced onions

3 garlic cloves, crushed

2 celery sticks, chopped

225 g diced carrots

1 small parsnip, diced small

1 tsp salt

¼ tsp nutmeg

225 g green split peas, rinsed and soaked for 8–10 hours and then drained

1.5 litres stock (see page 58)

⅛ tsp pepper

2 tbsp chopped fresh coriander

4 tbsp fresh parsley

— FAVA BEAN BRUSCHETTA —

PUT the fava beans, sun-dried tomatoes, garlic, salt and pepper in a blender to make a coarse purée. Heat oil in a frying pan, sauté broccoli with garlic and seasonings.

Lightly toast the bread, spread the bean mix and top it with sautéed broccoli. Serve warm, sprinkled with sesame seeds.

325 g cooked fava beans

4 tbsp sun-dried tomatoes

1 garlic clove, chopped

1 tbsp olive oil

450 g broccoli florets

2 garlic cloves, sliced

2 tbsp olive oil

4 slices country bread, cut into 2.5 cm slices

toasted sesame seeds, to sprinkle

sea salt and pepper

MAIN MEALS

— PENNE BAKE WITH BROCCOLI, SUN-DRIED TOMATOES AND CAPERS —

250–500 g of Italian penne
4 tbsp olive oil
4 tbsp breadcrumbs
3 garlic cloves, chopped
225 g purple broccoli, steamed
4 tbsp sun-dried tomatoes, chopped
2 tbsp capers
1 tsp chopped fresh rosemary
2 tbsp each chopped fresh parsley and basil

COOK the pasta in salted boiling water until *al dente*.

While the pasta is cooking, heat half the oil in a skillet over a low heat. Stir in breadcrumbs and cook, stirring until golden.

Add garlic and sauté for a few seconds before adding broccoli, chopped sun-dried tomatoes, capers and rosemary. Stir and cook until heated well. Season with salt and pepper.

Drain the pasta and quickly add to the skillet. Add remaining oil and herbs. Mix well and serve warm over a bed of winter greens or steamed Swiss chard.

— CORN BREAD WITH SAUTÉED VEGETABLES —

225 g corn meal
100 g barley flour
100 g oat flour
½ tsp salt
1 tsp baking powder
450 ml soy milk
1 tbsp apple concentrate or maple syrup

PREHEAT oven to 180°C/350°F/Gas Mark 4. Sift the dry ingredients together. Add milk and sweetener to dry ingredients and allow the mixture to stand for 1 hour. Next, bake in a greased loaf pan for 40–45 minutes. When cooked, cool it slightly on a wire rack before slicing. The corn bread squares can be brushed with olive oil and grilled briefly before serving.

HEAT the oil in a wok. Add leeks and onions with peeled garlic clove. Sauté until slightly soft, then discard the garlic clove. Stir in mushrooms, cauliflower and squash. Toss and sauté for 5–8 minutes. Add beansprouts and snow peas. Sauté for 2 minutes. Add all seasonings. Mix well and serve with warm corn bread.

For the sautéed vegetables:
2 tbsp sesame oil
100 g leeks, cut into matchsticks
100 g sliced onion
1 garlic clove, peeled
4–8 shiitake mushrooms, soaked, washed and thinly sliced
225 g cauliflower florets
225 g finely sliced squash
225 g beansprouts
225 g snow peas
1 tsp ground coriander
1 tbsp tamari sauce
1 tsp sugar

— WINTER VEGETABLES IN ORIENTAL SAUCE —

PREHEAT oven to 200°C/400°F/Gas Mark 6. Oil parsnips, swede and yam and roast in a hot oven until soft and golden. In a pan of salted water, cook the sprouts until bright in colour. Drain. Steam or quickly boil the carrots.

To assemble, mix the vegetables with the warm sauce over a low heat. Cook gently for 6–8 minutes or longer. Serve with sprinkled fresh herbs and warm bread.

4 tbsp olive oil
3 parsnips, cut into chunks
1 swede, cut in small chunks
2 yams or sweet potatoes, cut into chunks
10–12 Brussels sprouts, with hard leaves removed
3 carrots, cut into chunks

For the sauce:
2 tbsp olive oil
225 g chopped onions
1 tbsp grated root ginger
225 g cooked black-eyed beans,
partially mashed
450 g chopped tomatoes
4 tbsp chopped fresh coriander
450 ml coconut milk
1 tbsp soy sauce (optional)
sea salt and pepper

HEAT oil in a heavy pan and sauté onions and ginger until lightly brown. Add mashed beans to the onions together with salt and pepper. Next, stir in chopped tomatoes and mix well and cook for 5–6 minutes. Add half the chopped coriander, coconut milk and soy, if using. Stir well. Cover the pan and simmer for 5–6 minutes. Remove from heat and add remaining coriander.

— CAULIFLOWER IN BÉCHAMEL SAUCE WITH HERBED BAKED POTATOES —

For the Béchamel Sauce:
1 litre soy milk
6–8 mushrooms, chopped
½ pumpkin, diced
2 celery sticks, chopped
1 leek, chopped
4 garlic cloves, chopped
2 bay leaves
1 large onion, chopped
a little nutmeg
4 tbsp flour
chopped fresh herbs
sea salt and pepper

SIMMER the milk with all the vegetables for ½ hour. Keep it on a very low heat to avoid burning.

Heat oil on a low heat, stir in the flour and cook, stirring for a few minutes. The aroma of cooking flour will be released. Strain milk through a sieve and add to the flour in a thin stream, stirring constantly. Discard vegetables. Whisk vigorously and the sauce will thicken. Keep the sauce warm over a double broiler. Season to taste.

For the Cauliflower:
1 small head cauliflower
6–8 whole shallots
chopped fresh parsley, to sprinkle

STEAM the cauliflower and shallots briefly. Set them in a baking dish, pour the béchamel sauce all over and slightly brown under a grill. Sprinkle over fresh parsley. Serve warm with baked potatoes (recipe over).

Boil the potatoes whole for 8–10 minutes. Cook and peel and cut into quarters. Put the potatoes in a baking dish. Pour oil over, sprinkle with the rosemary and garlic and cook until brown in a preheated oven at 230°C/450°F/Gas Mark 8 for 25–30 minutes. Serve with the rest of the menu.

For the Herbed Baked Potatoes:
6 large potatoes
olive oil
fresh rosemary sprigs
6 whole garlic cloves

– POTATO AND COURGETTES RÖSTI WITH SAUTÉED ARTICHOKES AND MUSHROOMS –

Over a moderate heat, fry onion in one tablespoon of oil until soft. In a bowl, combine grated potatoes, courgettes and fried onions. Season with salt, pepper and herbs.

Heat the remaining oil in a pan and add potato mixture. Cook for 6–8 minutes, stirring occasionally. Next, flatten the mix into a cake form and cook until browned and cooked through – about 8–10 minutes. The top of the cake can also be browned under a grill.

Serve it hot and cut into wedges.

3 tbsp olive oil
225 g chopped onion
4–5 potatoes, peeled and coarsely grated
2 courgettes, coarsely grated
4 tbsp chopped fresh parsley
sea salt and pepper

Heat two tablespoons of oil in a frying pan and sauté mushrooms, artichokes and shallots until golden. Remove from pan and keep them warm.

Place garlic, capers and herbs in a mortar and mash into a paste or use a food processor. Whisk mustard, salt, pepper and remaining olive oil into the garlic and caper mix. Mix well. Pour this sauce over mushrooms and artichokes.

Oil a gratin dish and arrange artichokes and mushrooms in it. Mix with tomato slices in alternate layers and sprinkle with a little lemon juice. Grill for 10–15 minutes before serving.

For the artichokes and
mushrooms:
6 tbsp olive oil
675 g sliced mushrooms
8 cooked artichoke hearts, sliced
2 shallots, chopped
2 garlic cloves, crushed
2 tbsp capers
2 tbsp chopped fresh chervil
2 tbsp chopped fresh parsley
100 g chopped fresh basil
2 tbsp mustard
tomato slices
lemon juice
sea salt and pepper

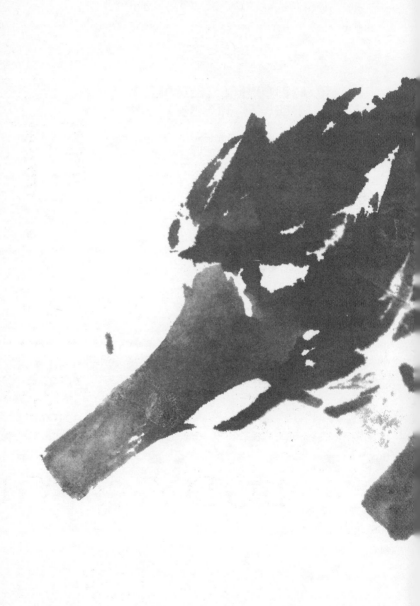

SECTION | **III**

....

HARMONY
BETWEEN
BODY & SOUL

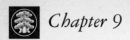

Chapter 9

Meditation – The Art of Inner Gardening

In the West we do not practise meditation because we too readily dismiss it as being part and parcel of a lifestyle which is impossible to integrate with our own. Ascetic spirituality seems an incoherent ideal in the everyday mode of family, work and the need to sustain social life. We have notions that meditation is something that Indian *sadhus* or Zen monks practise in far-away lands, cloistered away from the world and its need of us. And yet it is today that we need meditation perhaps far more than in the times of Buddha or the other venerable Indian masters who taught the importance of silence, and of looking at the world as though into a looking-glass that reflects back images of ourselves.

The Bible tells us that paradise is a garden. We may deduce that a good path to that paradise is the creation of our own gardens, not just physical places to grace our homes, but an inner space, a sanctuary where we find enchantment and regeneration that is entirely our own. This is a place where we come to take a rest from all those hooks that anchor us to life – stress, grief, worry, anger, frustration – and allow them to be dissolved and transformed into more positive, workable energy patterns. The garden is also the magical seat where

feelings that give us wings to fly through life – joy, compassion, enthusiasm, love, friendship – are enhanced and valued. And, lastly, the garden is also a place of silence and stillness, where only the pulsing of our being is felt. If we have never had any experience of soul, this is where the meeting is finally going to happen. Meditation is the art of inner gardening.

> Sitting silently,
> Doing nothing,
> Spring comes,
> And the grass grows by itself.
> – Osho, *Talks on Zen*

CREATING THE INNER GARDEN

Meditation is very simple; all you need is the wish to enter a wondrous journey, a cushion to sit on and a place where you feel safe, relaxed and private. Visit the rooms in your home and find a spot where you feel that you can begin creating the inner garden. It may be a room which is not used very frequently, somewhere you can retire to and feel that you can be alone and silent. This spot may change at different times of the year – you may be drawn to meditate outdoors in late spring and summer, or that you need a warmer spot in winter.

Although initially this may be diffi-cult, it is best to meditate every day for forty-five minutes to one hour. Entering the inner garden is like passing through a mystical gate, and things are not the same on the other side, thus it takes a little time to adjust to the different climate. Be patient, you will soon begin to reap the benefits from your hour alone cultivating the inner garden.

The best times for meditation are early morning and evening and these are the hours where consciousness is most transparent; if you meditate between 6–7 am, and 7–8 pm, you will find it easier to be completely immersed in the silence of your being. Dawn and dusk are especially magical times, when the quality of light is between day and night, suffusing the world with softness. It is very beautiful to be still when everything around is slowly stirring to awaken or settling down to rest.

We now outline some simple and yet powerful meditations that anyone can practise; we suggest you read all the med-itations given in the following sections and then choose one that most appeals to you. Practise this one meditation every day for a minimum of three weeks to three months. If you find it helpful, keep a med-itation journal and observe the changes as they unfold. You may want to start your meditation course on a particular day, such as on the new moon, full moon or at an equinox. These are cosmically charged times and the energies whirling around you will help to focus your attention on the meditative process. Meditation is not an heroic act – it is about the deep, mysterious stirrings of your being. You may be disappointed at first and feel that nothing is happening to you. Do not as a consequence become obsessed and practise

as though you were muscle-building. Be patient. Be still and know. The changes that will happen may not be great, but they will be profound and will alter the quality of other areas of your life.

The following meditations were devised or adapted from ancient methods by Osho, an enlightened master who has been working with all possibilities to help humanity develop and raise consciousness. His established commune in Pune, India, and his many centres all over the world help thousands to experience meditation and transformation. His teachings have influenced millions of people of all ages and from all walks of life.

VIPASSANA

Find a comfortable place to sit for 45 to 60 minutes. It helps to sit at the same time and in the same place every day, and it doesn't have to be a silent place. Experiment until you find the situation you feel best in. You can sit once or twice a day, but don't sit for at least an hour after eating or before sleeping.

It's important to sit with your back and head straight. Your eyes should be closed and your body as still as possible. A meditation bench can help, or a straight-backed chair or any arrangement of cushions.

There is no special breathing technique; ordinary, natural breathing is fine. Vipassana is based on the awareness of the breath, so the rise and fall of each breath should be watched, wherever the sensation is felt most clearly – at the nose or in the area of the stomach or solar plexus.

Vipassana is not concentration and it is not an objective to remain watching the breathing for a whole hour. When thoughts, feelings or sensations arise, or when you become aware of sound, smells and breezes from outside, simply allow the attention to go to them. Whatever comes up can be watched as clouds passing in the sky – you neither cling nor reject.

Whenever there is a choice of what to watch, return to awareness of breathing.

Remember, nothing special is meant to happen. There is neither success nor failure – nor is there any improvement. There is nothing to figure out or analyse, but insights may come about anything. Questions and problems may be just seen as mysteries to be enjoyed.

– Osho, from *The Revolution*

NADABRAHMA

Nadabrahma is an old Tibetan technique which was originally done in the early hours of the morning. It can be done at any time of the day, alone or with others, but have an empty stomach and remain inactive for at least fifteen minutes afterwards. The meditation lasts an hour and there are three stages. You may apply for the Nadabrahma meditation tape, with different music announcing each stage, at the addresses given in the appendix section of meditation tapes and music.

First stage: thirty minutes
Sit in a relaxed position with eyes closed and lips together. Start humming, loudly enough to be heard by others and create a vibration throughout your body. You can visualize a hollow tube or an empty vessel, filled only with the vibrations of the humming. A point will come when the humming continues by itself and you become the listener. There is no special breathing and you can alter the pitch or move your body smoothly and slowly if you feel like it.

Second stage: fifteen minutes
The second stage is divided into two 7½ minute sections. For the first half, move the hands, palms up, in an outward circular

motion. Starting at the navel, both hands move forwards and then divide to make two large circles mirroring each other left and right. The movement should be so slow that at times there will appear to be no movement at all. Feel that you are giving energy outwards to the universe.

After 7½ minutes turn the hands, palms down, and start moving them in the opposite direction. Now the hands will come together towards the navel and divide outwards to the sides of the body. Feel that you are taking energy in. As in the first stage, don't inhibit any soft, slow movements of the rest of your body.

Third stage: fifteen minutes
Sit absolutely quiet and still.

– Osho, from *Meditation: The First and Last Freedom*

NADABRAHMA FOR COUPLES

Osho has given a beautiful variation of this technique for couples.
Partners sit facing each other, covered by a bed-sheet and holding each other's crossed hands. It is best to wear no other clothing.

Light the room only by four small candles, and burn a particular incense, kept only for this meditation.

Close your eyes and hum together for thirty minutes. After a short while the energies will be felt to meet, merge and unite.

– Osho, from *Meditation: The First and Last Freedom*

SHIVA NETRA

This third-eye meditation is in two stages, repeated three times – a total of six 10-minute stages.
First stage: ten minutes
Sit perfectly still and, with eyes softly focussed, watch a blue light.

Second Stage: ten minutes
   Close your eyes and slowly and gently sway from side to side.

Repeat three times.

   – Osho, from *The Orange Book*

PRAYER MEDITATION

It is best to do this prayer at night, in a darkened room, going to sleep immediately afterwards; or it can be done in the morning, but it must be followed by fifteen minutes rest. This rest is necessary, otherwise you will feel as if you are drunk, in a stupor.
   This merging with energy is prayer. It changes you. And when you change, the whole existence changes.
   Raise both your hands towards the sky, palms uppermost, head up, just feeling existence flowing in you.
   As the energy flows down your arms you will feel a gentle tremor – be like a leaf in a breeze, trembling. Allow it, help it. Then let your whole body vibrate with energy, and just let whatever happens happen.
   You feel again a flowing with the earth. Earth and heaven, above and below, yin *and* yang, *male and female – you float, you mix, you drop yourself completely. You are not. You become one...merge.*
   After two to three minutes, or whenever you feel completely filled, lean down to the earth and kiss the earth. You simply become a vehicle to allow the divine energy to unite with that of the earth.
   These two stages should be repeated six more times so that each of the chakras can become unblocked. More times can be done, but if you do less you will feel restless and unable to sleep. Go into sleep in that very state of prayer. Just fall asleep and the energy will be there. You
will *be flowing with it, falling into sleep.*
   That will help very greatly because then the energy will surround you the whole night and it will continue to work. By the morning you will feel more fresh than you have ever felt before, more vital than you have ever felt before. A new élan, a new life will start penetrating you, and the whole day you will feel full of new energy; a new vibe, a new song in your heart, and a new dance in your step.
   – Osho, from *Meditation: The First and Last Freedom*

GOURISHANKAR

This technique consists of four stages of fifteen minutes each. The first two stages prepare the meditator for the spontaneous Latihan of the third stage. Osho has said that if the breathing is done correctly in the first stage the carbon dioxide formed in the bloodstream will make you feel as high as Gourishankar (Mount Everest).
First stage: fifteen minutes
   Sit with closed eyes. Inhale deeply through the nose, filling the lungs. Hold the breath for as long as possible, then exhale gently through the mouth and keep the lungs empty for as long as possible. Continue this breathing cycle throughout the first stage.

Second stage: fifteen minutes
   Return to normal breathing and with a gentle gaze look at a candle flame or a flashing blue light. Keep your body still.

Third stage: fifteen minutes
   With closed eyes, stand up and let your body be loose and receptive. The subtle energies will be felt to move the body outside your normal control. Allow this Latihan to happen. Don't do the moving: let the moving happen, gently and gracefully.

Fourth stage: fifteen minutes

Lie down with your eyes closed, silent and still.

– Osho, from *Meditation: The First and Last Freedom*

The first three stages should be accompanied by a steady rhythmic beat, preferably combined with a soothing background music. The beat should be seven times the normal heartbeat and, if possible, the flashing light should be a synchronised strobe. You can purchase the music tape for Gourishankar from the retailers listed in the appendix section of meditation tapes and music.

MIRROR-GAZING MEDITATION

This is the meditation to uncover your original face. It lasts forty minutes. You will need a mirror and a candle. Practise in a darkened room.

Close the doors of your room and put a big mirror just in front of you. The room must be dark. And then put a small flame by the side of the mirror in such a way that is not directly reflected in it. Just your face is reflected in the mirror, not the flame. Then constantly stare into your own eyes in the mirror. Do not blink. This is a forty-minute experiment, and within two or three days you will be able to keep your eyes unblinking.

Even if tears come, let them come, but persist in not blinking and go on staring constantly into your eyes. Do not change the stare. Go on staring into the eyes, your own, and within two or three days you will become aware of a very strange phenomenon. Your face will begin to take new shapes. You may even be scared. The face in the mirror will begin to change.

Sometimes a very different face will be there

which you have never known as yours.

But, really, all these faces belong to you. Now the subconscious mind is beginning to explode. These faces, these masks, are yours. Sometimes even a face that belongs to a past life may come in. After one week of constant staring for forty minutes, your face will become a flux, just a film-like flux. Many faces will be coming and going constantly. After three weeks, you will not be able to remember which is your face. You will not be able to remember your own face, because you have seen so many faces coming and going.

If you continue, then any day, after three weeks, the most strange thing happens: suddenly there is no face in the mirror. The mirror is vacant, you are staring into emptiness. There is no face at all. This is the moment: close your eyes, and encounter the unconscious.

You will be naked – completely naked, as you are. All deceptions will fall.

– Osho, from *The Ultimate Alchemy, Vol. I*

THE UNWINDING MEDITATION

This is a meditation for those who practise at night, just before going to sleep.

As you lie in bed, waiting for sleep, take a few moments to unwind, literally. Start thinking of everything you have done that day in reverse order. Begin with 'I took a few moments to unwind. I got comfortable in bed. I went to bed. I put my pyjamas on…' and so on until you reach the moment you awoke that morning.

OFFICE MEDITATIONS

Office stress can be counteracted with simple, yet effective meditations; this is an intelligent way of taking care of yourself and to put an end to the pattern of receiving abuse through untoward situations that crop up in your work and of giving out abuse to others or to yourself. Be gentle, be patient, and find a way to disperse stress so that it does not harm you or others. Meditation in the office returns you to your wholeness and integrity.

GIBBERISH

This is a highly cathartic technique, which encourages expressive body movements.

Either alone or in a group, close your eyes and begin to say nonsense sounds – gibberish. For fifteen minutes move totally in the gibberish. Allow yourself to express whatever needs to be expressed within you.

Throw everything out. The mind thinks, always, in terms of words. Gibberish helps break up this pattern of continual verbalisation. Without suppressing your thoughts, you can throw them out – in gibberish. Let your body likewise be expressive.

Then, for fifteen minutes, lie down on your stomach and feel as if you are merging with mother earth. With each exhalation, feel yourself merging into the ground beneath you.

– Osho, from *The Orange Book*

PONDERING ON THE OPPOSITE

This is a beautiful method. It will be very useful. For example: if you are feeling very discontented, what to do? Ponder on the opposite. If you are feeling discontented, contemplate about contentment. What is contentment? Bring a balance. If your mind is angry, bring compassion in, think about compassion; and immediately the energy changes because they

are the same. The opposite is the same energy. Once you bring it in it absorbs. Anger is there, contemplate on compassion.

Do one thing: keep a statue of Buddha, because that statue is the gesture of compassion. Whenever you feel angry, go into the room, look at Buddha, sit Buddha-like and feel compassion. Suddenly you will see a transformation happening within you. The anger is changing: excitement gone, compassion arising. And it is not different energy – the same energy as anger – changing its quality, going higher. Try it!

– Osho, from *The Orange Book*

WRITING DOWN YOUR THOUGHTS

One day do this: a little experiment. Close your doors and sit in your room and just start writing your thoughts – whatsoever comes into your mind. Don't change them because you need not show this piece of paper to anybody! Just go on writing for ten minutes and then look at them. This is what your thinking is. If you look at them you will think this is some madman's work. If you show that piece of paper to your most intimate friend he will also look at you and think 'Have you gone crazy?'

– Osho, from *No Water, No Moon*

MEDITATION AND WORK

Whenever you feel that you are not in a good mood and you don't feel good in the work, before starting work, just for five minutes, exhale deeply. Feel with the exhalation that you are throwing your dark mood out and you will be surprised within five minutes you will be suddenly back to normal and the low will have disappeared, the dark is no more there.

– Osho, from *Don't Bite My Finger, Look Where I'm Pointing*

If you change your work into meditation,
that's the best thing. Then meditation is never
in conflict with your life. Whatsoever you do
can become meditative. Meditation is not some-
thing separate; it is a part of life. It is just
like breathing: just as you breathe in and out,
you meditate also.

And it is simply a shift of emphasis;
nothing much is to be done. Things that you
have been doing carelessly, start doing care-
fully. Things that you have been doing for
some results, for example, money...That's
okay, but you can make it a plus phenomenon.
Money is okay and if work gives you money,
good; one needs money, but it is not all. And
just by the side if you can reap many more
pleasures, why miss them? They are just free
of cost.

You will be doing your work whether you
love it or not, so just bringing love to it you
will reap many more things which otherwise
you would miss.

– Osho, from *Dance Your Way to God*

KITCHEN TEMPLE MEDITATION

Transform the time of preparing your meals
into your evening meditation. Chop vegetables
Zen-style. Be silent, concentrate on every move-
ment of your hands, one action at a time, all
the while breathing deeply in and out. Be slow
and careful. Honour the spirit of the ingredi-
ents you are chopping and thank existence for
providing you with beautiful abundance.

Chapter 10

A PRACTICAL

GUIDE TO

HEALTH FOODS

AND

SUPPLEMENTS

WHILE *it may be very difficult to strike personal relationships with the staff in a supermarket, one of the great joys of shopping in small stores is that you can have a one-to-one rapport with the people working there. This is especially so in health food stores, which are generally vision-led and where the employees have a keen and informed interest in the products they are selling. One can talk to them, ask for advice, exchange tips and generally cultivate a soulful relationship with the people one is buying food from. We suggest that you start visiting your local health food store and, while you are shopping, ask questions and acquire further knowledge of what you are buying. You should also find out where your nearest organic greengrocer is and whether it offers weekly home deliveries as this is a very convenient service. You can buy certain items, such as grains or carrots and apples for juicing, in bulk for long-term storing.*

Here we give you a brief summary and glossary of those items that appear in the recipes. Use this as a guide-

line, but we encourage you to experiment on your own and get acquainted with the products as you buy and use them.

GRAINS

GRAINS *play a fundamental part in any vegetarian diet – they are high in complex carbohydrates and low in fat and small quantities provide great nourishment. Grains are the staple food for the soul – they connect us to the Earth, enhance receptivity, relaxation and centredness. We suggest that you stock a few of your favourite grains in your pantry for the preparation of everyday meals. You may also want to invest in an electric rice cooker – a very convenient kitchen appliance that keeps a constant temperature and cooks all grains to perfection. The Japanese company Zojirushi makes excellent rice cookers in different sizes which are available from the bigger department stores in both Britain and the United States.*

– AMARANTH –

Benefits: lungs.
Cooking method: to 225 g grain add 550–675 ml of water (increasing water improves the tenderness of the cooked grain). Bring to the boil and simmer covered for 20–25 minutes.
Suggested use: sweet cereal, biscuits, casseroles, breads, soups; you can also sprout it and use it in salads.

THIS is a relatively new discovery in the family of grains, even though amaranth is of very ancient origin – the Aztecs used it in their diets. It has a high nutritional value being a rich source of protein and calcium. Excellent during pregnancy and for nursing mothers as well as infants. It is best used in combination with other grains, such as wheat, to make it more palatable.

— BARLEY —

THIS ancient grain has been used throughout the centuries for its nourishing properties. Barley is milled to remove the indigestible hull. There are two varieties: pearl barley and pot (also known as Scotch) barley. Pearl barley has been processed to remove both the germ and the chaff during milling, thus removing some of the nutritional value. Pot barley is a rich source of fibre, calcium and iron. Pot barley is often toasted before cooking to reduce its acid-forming qualities.

Benefits: stomach, spleen, pancreas.

Cooking method: to 225g of grain add 675 ml–1 litre of water, bring to the boil and simmer covered for 50–55 minutes.

Suggested use: breads, cereals, crackers, soups and stews. Decoction of barley water is very good for convalescents.

— BUCKWHEAT/KASHI —

THIS grain is widely used in eastern Europe, China and Japan. It is well-recognised for containing an almost perfect natural balance of amino acids, as well as providing calcium and proteins. The buckwheat plant seems to resist the attack of many diseases and can thus grow naturally without the aid of pesticides. When it is toasted it is called *kashi*. This is a grain that produces heartiness and helps the body keep warm, so it is perfect for the chilly days of winter.

Benefits: intestines (not recommended for people with high blood pressure or wind).

Cooking method: rinse it well under cold water and toast it. To 225g of grain add 450 ml of water, bring to the boil and simmer covered for 15–20 minutes.

Suggested use: pancakes, stuffings, pasta or noodles, cereal bread.

— BULGAR WHEAT —

THIS grain belongs to the wheat family and is obtained from boiled, dried and cracked wheat berries. It is rich in fibre, minerals and vitamins, providing a wide range of nutritional qualities essential for growth and well-being. It is best used in its organic, unrefined form.

Benefits: kidneys.

Cooking method: to 225 g of grain add 450 ml of boiling water, cover and allow it to stand for 30 minutes (no need to cook it). Fluff it with a fork.

Suggested use: pilaffs, salads, stuffings.

— CRACKED WHEAT —

THIS grain has the same nutritional qualities as bulgar wheat. To release its flavour, toast it until fragrant.

Cooking method: to 225 g of grain add 675 ml of boiling water, bring to the boil and simmer covered for 35–40 minutes.
Suggested use: soft cereals, salads, casseroles.

— CORN(MAIZE) —

THIS is a grain which is widely cultivated throughout the world from Italy (polenta) and the rest of Europe to Asian countries and North America. It is also a staple of many African diets. Fresh corn (corn-on-the-cob) contains many vitamins and enzymes and is light enough to eat in the warm seasons. Because of its low niacin content, it is recommended to use corn in combination with wheatgerm, peanuts, brewer's yeast or lime juice.

Benefits: heart and kidney.
Cooking method: use a dry heat to make popcorn. 3 tbsp of corn makes 1.35 kg of pop corn. Use a non-stick pan with a lid. Boil the cobs and roast them if you want it fresh.
Suggested use: bread, dumplings (gnocchi), polenta (using the flour), corn tortillas, nachos, salads.

— MILLET —

A staple grain of India, Egypt and China, it has also been used throughout the centuries in Europe. In the tale *Hansel and Gretel*, little Hansel leaves a trail of millet grains to mark his way home from the depths of the dangerous forest, but the birds eat them and the two siblings get lost and end up in the witch's house. This is the only grain that causes no acidic reaction in the stomach whatever. It is well-known for its anti-fungal properties and is highly recommended for those who suffer from candida infections. It is very easily digested.

Benefits: stomach, spleen, pancreas.
Cooking method: toast first. To 225g of grain add 550 ml of boiling water. Bring to the boil and simmer covered for 35–40 minutes.
Suggested use: sweetened cereals, stews, casseroles, stuffings, breads and pancakes.

— OATS —

THIS is the ideal grain for cold weather and is widely used in the everyday diets of cold regions such as the Scottish Highlands (porridge) and Switzerland (it is the main component of muesli). Oats are a rich source of protein, as well as silicon and a variety of minerals, including iron. Whole oats have retained both the bran and the germ, where most nutritional qualities reside. Oats are immensely helpful in regulating energy swings and in calming the nerves.

Benefits: spleen, pancreas, nerves.
Cooking method: use organic whole oats. To 225g of grain add 675 ml of water. Soak overnight. Bring to the boil and simmer for 45–60 minutes. For rolled oats: to 225g of grain add 325 ml of water, stir, bring to the boil and cook for 10 minutes. Remove from heat and let it stand for 15 minutes.

— QUINOA —

IT belongs to the amaranth family and was a staple grain in the diet of the Incas. It is rich in protein and calcium and it is a strengthening grain for the whole body. This is an ideal food for those switching from a meat-eating to a vegetarian diet as it is packed with all of the necessary nutrients.

Benefits: kidneys.
Cooking method: to 225g grain add 450 ml of water, bring to the boil and simmer covered for 15 minutes.
Suggested use: salads, patties, breads, stuffings.

– RICE –

Varieties: organic, whole basmati rice is the lightest variety and is recommended for all stagnant conditions (water retention, etc.). Sweet rice is rich in gluten and high in protein and fat. Sprouted rice is a common herb prescribed by Chinese doctors.

Benefits: stomach, spleen, pancreas.

Cooking method: Long grain – to 225 g grain add 325 ml of boiling water, bring to the boil and simmer covered for 15–20 minutes.

Short grain – as above.

Brown basmati – to 225 g grain add 500 ml of water, bring to the boil and simmer covered for 35–40 minutes.

White basmati – to 225 g grain add 400 ml of water, bring to the boil and simmer covered for 20 minutes.

Sweet rice – to 225 g grain add 325 ml of water, bring to the boil and simmer covered for 55–60 minutes.

THIS is the staple grain in the modern world, eaten daily throughout Asia; its ancient origins are to be found in India, China and Japan. It has legendary healing powers and has for a long time been associated with Zen Buddhist rituals and traditions. Rice plays a key role in maintaining the flow of life energy in the body. We recommend you eat rice at least three times a week. It is a rich source of vitamin B and it has soothing properties for the nervous system. White rice is consumed more widely than brown rice, but the latter retains all of its nutrients and goodness as it is unrefined. Short grain varieties have a nuttier flavour.

— RYE —

THIS is a bitter-flavoured grain, highly recommended to reduce conditions of dampness in the body and benefits stagnancy in the liver and gall bladder. It contains considerable levels of fluoride which is essential for building enamel in teeth. Rye is a hard grain suited to harsh, cold climates and is mainly used for breads and biscuits.

Benefits: liver, spleen, gall bladder.
Suggested use: sourdough bread; when sprouted can be used in salads.
Cooking method: used mainly in flour form.

— WHEAT —

THIS is perhaps the most cultivated grain in the Western hemisphere as it is packed with nutrients when used in its unrefined form. Builds *yin* energy and is beneficial for the heart and mind. It is a rich source of minerals vitamins and fibre, promoting growth and health. Wheat berries and bulgar come from the same family. Wheat is known to cause allergic reactions in some people, in which case it is best avoided or substituted with rye or another cereal.

Benefits: kidneys, nerves.
Cooking method: mostly used in flour form for breads.
Wheat berries – soak overnight; to 225 g of grain add 750 ml of water, bring to the boil and simmer covered for 1 hour.

— WILD RICE —

ALTHOUGH used as rice, this is actually the wild seed of an aquatic grass which is now commonly used as a grain. It is closely related to corn and originates from North America. Wild rice provides high quality protein, vitamins, minerals and fibre. It is both cooling and diuretic.

Benefits: kidneys, bladder.
Cooking method: to 225g wild rice 750 ml of boiling water, bring to the boil and simmer covered for 1 hour.

LEGUMES

LEGUMES *and beans provide a substantial amount of protein in a vegetarian diet and should be incorporated in at least half of your weekly meals. It is best to use organic legumes, rather than the non-organic or tinned varieties. However, this means that time will be spent cooking them as most beans take one hour or more to be cooked. We suggest you invest in a pressure cooker which considerably reduces cooking time (generally by half) without decreasing any of the nutrients. Stock your pantry with a variety of legumes – they keep for months in sealed glass or plastic jars and can be eaten all year round. The longer you store the beans, the longer they will need to be cooked. Organic legumes tend to be harvested in the same year they are sold; check the dates on the packets and buy as fresh as possible. Follow our recipes for more elaborate dishes or serve freshly cooked beans in the colourful Mediterranean-style: with a drop of extra-virgin olive oil, a few leaves of basil, some salt and a topping such as black Greek olives, sun-dried tomatoes or strips of roasted red and green pepper.*

– ADUKI BEANS –

Cooking method: soak overnight. To 225g beans add 1 litre of water, bring to the boil and simmer covered for 1 hour.

ORIGINALLY from Asia, they are now widely available. They are one of the most digestible beans and particularly good for people with weak kidneys. Aduki beans are best flavoured with sea vegetables, shoyu sauce, spring onions, ginger, miso, garlic and pepper. They combine well with millet and the different varieties of rice.

— BLACK BEANS —

WIDELY used in Latin America and Asia. They are diuretic and build *yin* energy. They are best combined with rice or corn. Many seasonings go well with black beans: onions, fresh chopped tomatoes, green peppers, garlic, lemon juice and fresh herbs.

Cooking method: soak overnight. To 225 g beans add 1 litre water, bring to the boil and simmer covered for 1½ –2 hours.

— BLACK-EYED BEANS —

ORIGINALLY a wild species from Africa, they are now common in Western countries. They are a rich source of selenium. Quick to cook and easy to flavour, they are wonderful in salads, with sautéed spinach and combine well with many other seasonal vegetables.

Cooking method: no pre-soaking required. To 225g of beans add 1 litre of water, bring to the boil and simmer covered for 1–1½ hours.

— FAVA BEANS —

SWEET-FLAVOURED beans with a tough exterior skin which can be removed after soaking them overnight. This is a hearty bean used to strengthen the spleen and pancreas. Easily seasoned with onions, fresh chopped tomatoes, herbs and spices. Used to make stews, salads and pâtés.

Cooking method: soak overnight and remove outer skin before cooking. To 225 g of beans add 1 litre of water, bring to the boil and simmer covered for 1½ hours.

— CHICKPEAS —

THESE are perhaps the most popular beans in the Middle East, Asia, Africa and the Mediterranean countries. Chickpeas are a rich source of iron and unsaturated fat. Easy to use on their own or combined with vegetables and grains. Cumin, coriander, lemon juice, curry powder or simply olive oil with parsley are excellent flavourings for dressing these beans.

Cooking method: soak overnight. To 225 g of beans add 1 litre of water, bring to the boil and simmer covered for 2½ –3 hours.

— KIDNEY BEANS —

Cooking method: soak overnight. To 225 g of beans add 1 litre of water, bring to the boil and simmer covered for 1½ –2 hours.

BELONG to a large family of beans which includes pinto, green wax and mung beans. They are cooling and diuretic, but are perhaps the hardest beans to digest, even though they are easy to cook. Chilli and hot flavours combine well, as well as onion, garlic, coriander and other Eastern spices.

— LENTILS —

Cooking method: no pre-soaking required. To 225g lentils add 1 litre of water and cook for 30–35 minutes.

THERE are red, yellow, Puy and brown lentils. In European countries, they are a symbol of good luck and it is traditional in Germany to eat them on New Year's Eve. They are easy to cook and combine well with many grains and vegetables. Use ginger, onions, bay leaf, a tomato sauce or peppers to flavour them.

— LIMA BEANS —

Cooking method: soak overnight. To 225g of beans add 1 litre of water, bring to the boil and simmer covered for 1–1½ hours.

ALSO commonly known as butter beans; cooling and nourishing, easy to cook, they are particularly good for the liver and lungs. They have a high alkaline content and help combat acidity in the stomach. They go well with herbs such as fresh dill, parsley and basil. Excellent for making creamy soups.

— MUNG BEANS —

Cooking method: no pre-soaking required. To 225 g of beans add 1 litre of water, bring to the boil and simmer covered for 45–60 minutes.

THESE are the king beans of Zen food. Cooling, sweet-flavoured beans, well-known for their detoxifying properties, they increase *yin* energy. They are also available in their sprouted variety and can be added to salads and stir-fries. Good seasonings are: onion, ginger, coriander, tomato and even yoghurt.

— NAVY BEANS —

Sweet, cooling beans, most commonly used in baked beans. Their creamy texture goes well with such seasonings as onion, mustard or tomato sauce.

Cooking method: soak overnight. To 225g of beans add 1 litre of water, bring to the boil and simmer covered for 1½ –2 hours.

— DRIED PEAS —

There are two varieties – green and yellow. They are easy to digest and mildly diuretic. Good seasonings are: onion, bay leaf, turmeric or celery and they combine well with many vegetables.

Cooking method: no pre-soaking required. To 225g of beans add 1 litre of water. Bring to the boil and simmer for 1½ –2 hours.

— PINTO BEANS —

They take a long time to cook, but they hold their shape and are full of flavour. Used in many Mexican dishes, pinto beans combine well with onion, peppers, garlic, avocado and cumin.

Cooking method: soak overnight. To 225g of beans add 1 litre of water, bring to the boil and simmer covered for 2½ –3 hours.

— SOY BEANS —

Cooling and full of nutrients, soy beans are the base component of many soy products – tempeh, tofu, miso, shoyu. They need to be well cooked in order to be digested and are a high source of protein.

Cooking method: soak overnight. To 225g of beans add 1 litre of water. Bring to the boil and simmer covered for 2½ –3 hours.

— TIPS TO IMPROVE THE DIGESTIBILITY OF LEGUMES —

- Legumes combine best with greens and non-starchy vegetables and sea vegetables.
- Salt or salty seasonings should only be added at the end of the cooking time, so as not to toughen the skins. Salt is needed as it aids the digestion of the protein in beans.
- Cook legumes with cumin, fennel seeds, or a little vinegar to avoid forming gaseous reactions.
- Add kombu or kelp at the bottom of the pan to improve digestibility and add flavouring.
- Soak legumes overnight. A little flour helps soften the outer skins. Wash them well and never cook them in the soaking water.
- When boiling, remember to discard the foam that forms on the surface of the water.
- Sprouted legumes contain just as much protein and can be added to salads or stir-fries. Steam sprouts for better digestibility.

SOY PRODUCTS

— MISO —

Suggested use: as a salt substitute. Add to soups, stews, dressings, dips and gravies. Miso soup should be added to a vegetarian diet at least three to four times a week.

A paste made from fermented soy beans, barley or rice, each type having a distinctive colour and flavour. The red, dark varieties of miso are fermented longer and are best suited for the cold winter months. The lighter varieties are better for warmer weather. Miso is a live food, containing the bacteria *lactobacillus* that helps the digestive process, as well as protein and amino acids in the same pattern as in meat. Always buy unpasteurised miso and add to food during the last minutes, cooking minimally and never boiling in order not to kill its live bacteria. It is best to keep it stored in a glass jar in the refrigerator.

— TEMPEH —

COOKED and fermented soy beans, pounded into strips with herbs and seasonings. It is high in proteins, essential fats and fibre so it is a very nutritious food for vegetarians. It can be bought fresh, dried, pre-cooked or frozen in many health food stores. It can be steamed, fried or broiled.

Suggested use: pre-cooked tempeh is excellent in sandwiches. Also in kebabs, breads, burgers, stuffings, salads or stir-fries.

— TOFU —

THIS is a curd made from processed soy beans which have been soaked, cooked and blended in various stages. Tofu is a staple product of the Orient and it is widely used in China, Japan and Korea. Contains easily digestible proteins, vitamin B and minerals. It is low in calories and very satisfying to the palate. There are three basic types of tofu: silken, which is very soft; medium and firm tofu. The most commonly used is firm tofu which can be smoked, deep fried, frozen or marinated. Though rather bland in its original form, tofu easily absorbs other flavours. Those suffering from dairy-derived allergies can make many creamy desserts and dressings from tofu. Store in a cool place in an airtight container.

Suggested use: casseroles, thick sauces, stir-fries, salads, scrambled, soups.

SEA VEGETABLES

SEA vegetables share the common characteristic of being one of the highest sources of vitamins and minerals, containing up to twenty times the minerals of land plants. They are literally a wonder food providing excellent dietary medicinal value as they detoxify, activate liver energy, alkalise the blood and are beneficial to the thyroid. They also have a calming effect on the nervous system when eaten regularly. Widely used in Japanese cuisine, sea vegetables are now sold in health food stores and oriental shops. We suggest you buy a few varieties and incorporate them into your meals at least six or seven times a week, either just soaked and lightly steamed in salads or cooked with tofu or grains.

Cooking method: always rinse sea vegetables thoroughly before using. Dry sea vegetables should be soaked before cooking – longer soaking makes them more tender. Fresh sea vegetables can be sautéed lightly or used in salads.

— AGAR AGAR —

THIS is a gelatine-like sea vegetable that can be bought in either powder or flake form. Soften flakes or dissolve powder in some water. Bring to the boil with some water, juice or broth, stirring constantly. Add the other ingredients of the recipe and set in moulds.

Suggested use: gelatine, aspic, kanten, mousses.

— ARAME —

THIS is one of the richest sources of iodine and is excellent for those suffering from high blood pressure or feminine disorders. Arame is a member of the kelp family.

Cooking method: Soak for 10 to 15 minutes as it expands in volume. Chop and cook with soups, stews or grains; sauté or steam lightly and add to salads.

— HIJIKI —

THIS is a rich source of iron, calcium and vitamin B2. Helps to keep blood sugar at optimum levels and has a calming effect on the nerves. It is full of flavour and can be used on its own as part of a main meal. Follow cooking instructions for arame.

— KANTEN —

THIS is a dish made from any ingredient which has been jellied with agar agar. For a delicious dessert use seasonal fruit, such as berries and peaches. Serve chilled.

— KOMBU AND KELP —

THESE are two marine plants full of the goodness of the sea; they benefit the kidneys, help balance the thyroid and their prolonged use also helps prevent arthritis and rheumatism. They both have a very high mineral content.

Cooking method: cut or break into bite-size pieces. Soak for 20–30 minutes in warm water. Add to boiling water and cook for 1–1½ hours. Roast it and ground it into a powder and sprinkle on salads. Also good to use in soups and stews. When added to cooking beans, it enhances their digestibility.

— NORI —

THIS is the seaweed wrapped around Japanese *sushi*. Known for its high protein content, nori grows as a large flat plant and is bought in packets containing thin sheets, folded into four. The easiest way to prepare it is to hold it over a live flame, toasting it slowly until it changes colour to a darker shade of green. Can be used in *sushi* or cut into strips and sprinkled over salads, soups and grains. It promotes the digestion of fried food.

— WAKAME —

IN Japan, it is used to purify blood. As with other sea vegetables, it is a rich source of calcium and niacin and promotes healthy, beautiful skin and hair. Soak for 3–4 minutes, drain, cut into strips and cut the tough mid-rib. Cook in boiling water for 45 minutes. Use in soups, stews or with grains.

STOCKING YOUR PANTRY

HERE we list a few items that are the staples of a healthy pantry and used in the preparation of many recipes. You will find of all these items in a well-stocked health food store and some larger supermarkets may carry one or two of these products. Clearspring Wholefoods is a company which distributes excellent organic products and imports the original items from countries such as Japan.

— ARROWROOT —

THIS is a starch flour used as a thickening agent. Dissolve in water before adding to the dish you are preparing.

— BANCHA TEA —

ALSO known as *kuki-cha,* this tea comes from Japan and is drunk as a healthy, refreshing breakfast beverage. It helps improve digestion.

— BARLEY MALT —

THIS is a sweetener made from barley and corn and can be used instead of sugar when preparing desserts.

— BLACK SESAME SEEDS —

SMALL black seeds to sprinkle over salads and grains for flavour. They are one of the highest sources of calcium.

— BOK CHOY —

A leafy Chinese vegetable belonging to the cabbage family. It has thick white stems that turn into dark green leaves. Used mainly in summer.

— BROWN RICE VINEGAR —

A very mild vinegar made from fermented brown rice. Ideal in salad dressings.

— DAIKON —

A long and quite large white radish used extensively in Japanese cuisine. It can be bought in oriental supermarkets or health food stores. Grated daikon aids the digestion of oily food.

— GINGER ROOT —

THIS is a pungent root which is widely used as a seasoning in many recipes. We recommend you buy fresh organic ginger.

— GOMASIO —

THIS is a seasoning made from ground sesame seeds and sea salt, it is a very good source of minerals and can be used instead of salt or sprinkled over grains and salads.

— GRAIN COFFEE —

YOU may choose a non-caffeine variety made from either organic barley or dandelion – these are warming drinks for cold winter mornings and afternoons.

— KUZU —

A white starch made from the root of the wild kuzu plant, used as a thickening for sauces, soups and desserts.

— SENCHA TEA —

THIS is the Japanese green tea favoured by Zen monks to promote mental clarity and calmness during meditation.

— SHIITAKE MUSHROOMS —

YOU may buy them either fresh-grown locally or dried-imported from Japan. They add a strong flavour to stocks and soups.

— SOBA NOODLES —

JAPANESE noodles made from buckwheat flour. Can be served either cold as a salad or hot with broth and vegetables.

— TAMARI SAUCE —

NATURALLY and organically made soy sauce obtained after two years of fermenting soy beans with sea salt.

— UDON —

JAPANESE wholewheat noodles, lighter than soba.

— UMEBOSHI —

PICKLED salted Japanese plums, which assist the digestive process by keeping the blood alkaline. Used for their medicinal properties, they are especially good in helping to detoxify the liver. They can be used with cooked vegetables, salads, in salad dressings or finely chopped on corn on the cob. The umeboshi water can be added to warm water and drank to relieve hangover and intestinal disorders. Umeboshi can be found in health food stores and in Japanese supermarkets.

— WASABI —

JAPANESE strong horseradish paste with a highly pungent flavour. Used in *sushi* and salad dressings.

HEALTH FOOD SUPPLEMENTS

THERE are two kinds of supplements: those derived from food or naturally available substances such as bee pollen or evening primrose oil and supplements which have been manufactured by man in order to complement lack of vitamins, minerals or amino acids. If we are healthy, happy, drink fresh raw juices, eat organic produce and follow a wholesome diet, meditate and exercise regularly, food-derived supplements should be sufficient to help us maintain an optimum degree of health. However, there may be times and conditions which need more careful examination and additional quantities of essential vitamins, minerals and amino acids.

Poor dietary patterns prolonged over time, chronic stress, hereditary conditions which severely affect the metabolism, chronic illness, extreme depression, pregnancy and breast-feeding – these are some of the most common areas which affect us physically, mentally and spiritually, causing a severe depletion of our resources. If you are experiencing any of these, we suggest you seek the guidance of an expert nutritionist who will help discern which supplements you need. Supplements of any sort should ideally be taken for a minimum period of three weeks to the optimal three months in order to feel the full benefits and in combination with a wholesome diet, meditation and exercise. Supplements, however, do not replace a healthy diet and lifestyle and should not be taken as staples – they help re-balance the system when there exists a deficiency, but should be decreased as the condition improves.

Here we list natural food supplements that can be safely added to your diet in order to maximise health and strengthen the immune system. When buying them, make sure that they are wholly natural organically grown, prepared without any additives and that they do not contain gelatine, dairy products or yeast. Health food stores stock all of these products and will help guide your choices.

— BREWER'S YEAST —

THIS is a plant without chlorophyll (which produces the green colouring in plants). It is an excellent source of B-complex vitamins as well as amino acids, protein, iron and copper. It is known to help maintain appetite, improve digestion, calm the nervous system and relieve anaemia. It is available in powder form, tablets or flakes. Those suffering from poor digestion benefit from it greatly, although they may feel bloating with large doses – start on a low dosage and progressively increase over the weeks.

— BEE POLLEN —

CONTAINS 35% protein, is high in B-complex vitamins and a rich source of lecithin. This is an ideal food supplement for vegans being a natural multi-vitamin and mineral supplement. Promotes emotional well-being, prevents colds and flu, has a beneficial effect upon the intestinal tract and is said to slow down the ageing process. It should be taken regularly up to 30 grams a day especially in the change from winter to spring. It is available in powder form, granules or tablets.

— CHLORELLA —

THIS is a freshwater alga and a concentrated source of easily digestible protein, as well as beta-carotene and nucleic acid which decreases with age, stress and pollution. Strengthens the immunity system, improves growth patterns and is extremely beneficial for anaemic conditions, chronic constipation and wind. It is available in powder form or tablets.

— CO Q10 —

CO-ENZYME Q10 was first discovered in 1957 as a substance present in the body, but not manufactured by it, so it needs to be supplemented by diet. Only recently introduced into the market, CO Q10 is a catalyst for releasing cell energy and when its level in the body drops by 25% degenerative conditions are set in motion. Healthy hearts have been found to have a high concentration of the co-enzyme. As well as strengthening the heart it is also a powerful antioxidant. Most people have an adequate supply of it and supplements should be taken in consultation with a nutritionist.

— EVENING PRIMROSE OIL —

THIS is an edible plant which stimulates the action of the stomach, helps lift depression and stimulates the spleen and liver. It helps control arthritis and blood pressure and is rich in potassium and magnesium. Evening primrose oil has long been hailed as the regulator of women's monthly cycles.

— GARLIC —

THIS common plant is a natural antibiotic. It dissolves cholesterol in the bloodstream, reduces blood pressure and helps detoxify. It is also a natural source of vitamins and minerals.

— GINKO BILOBA —

THIS is perhaps one of the most ancient trees alive on Earth today; it was worshipped by the early Buddhists for its strength and ability to survive for centuries. European studies show that ginko increases the flow of blood to the brain, thus reducing the ageing of its tissues. It has been found to have positive effects in treating asthma, memory decline, headaches and insomnia. Can be found in capsule form.

— GINSENG —

THIS is the king of herbs, used for centuries in Chinese medicine. It is a stimulant, relieving fatigue and stress. In Chinese medicine it is used as a general tonic for the mind, body and spirit and it can act as an antidote to the harmful effects of drugs and chemicals. It also contains vitamins A and E. It is available in tea form, in extract and capsules.

— KELP —

THIS is a sea vegetable and thus a rich source of minerals. It helps control thyroid activity, regulates the metabolism, strengthens the nervous system, promotes glandular health and is highly recommended during pregnancy. Available in tablet form.

— LECITHIN —

THIS is a substance found in our own cells, helping the transportation of fats to the different parts of the body and regulating the production of bile which is critical in fat production and absorption. It is also recommended as a stimulant of brain functions. Available in granules, capsules and liquid form.

— SPIRULINA —

THIS is an ancient food used by the Aztecs, although its wonderful properties have only been rediscovered recently. It is a blue-green micro-algae, packed with protein and minerals which are easily digestible. It has cleansing and detoxifying properties, especially for the liver; provides vitamins B12, A and E and is said to have a rejuvenating effect. Reduces food cravings, especially for animal protein. Available in tablet form.

— WILD BLUE-GREEN ALGAE —

THIS is a water plant that grows wild in the uncontaminated waters of Klamath Lake in the state of Oregon. Native American tribes regarded it to be the sister of the magic cactus peyote and used it for deepening meditation and trance states. Today, it is used to help detoxify, help concentration and clear away states of depression or melancholy. As its effects on the mind and body are very strong, use it in moderation, starting with a low dosage and progressively increasing to a medium dosage over a period of weeks.

APPENDIX

Tapes and CDs for some of the meditations outlined in Part II – *Harmony Between Body and Soul*, Chapter 9: 'The Art of Inner Gardening' can be obtained from the following addresses:

In the UK –

Osho International,
24 St. James's Street,
London SW1 1HA.
Telephone: 0171-925 1900
Fax: 0171-925 1901
E-mail: osho_int@osho.org

Osho Purnima,
'Greenwise',
Vange Park Road,
Basildon,
Essex
SS16 5LA.
Telephone: 01268-584141
Fax: 01268-559919

In the United States –

New Earth Records,
PO Box 2368,
Boulder CO 80306
Telephone: 800-570 4074

Osho America,
14305 North 79th Street,
PO Box 12517,
Scottsdale AZ 85260
Telephone: 602-905 2612
Fax: 602-905 2618
Orders: 800 777 7743
E-mail: osho_america@osho.org

BIBLIOGRAPHICAL REFERENCES

Blauer, S. *The Juicing Book.* New York: Avery Publishing Group, 1989

Colbin, A. *Food and Healing.* New York: Ballantine Books, 1986

Dogen and K. Uchiyama. *From the Zen Kitchen to Enlightenment.* New York and Tokyo: Weatherhill, 1994

Elson, M. Haas, MD. *Staying Healthy with the Seasons.* Berkeley: Celestial Arts, 1981

Kabat-Zinn, J. *Wherever You Go, There You Are.* New York: Hyperion, 1994

Kushi, M. *The Macrobiotic Way.* New York: Avery Publishing Group, 1993

Moore, T. *The Re-Enchantment of Everyday Life.* New York: HarperCollins, 1996

Osho. *Dance Your Way to God.* Pune, India: Rajneesh Foundation, 1978

—. *Don't Bite My Finger, Look Where I'm Pointing.* Rajneeshpuram, Oregon: Rajneesh Foundation International, 1982

—. *From Medication to Meditation.* Saffron Walden: C. W. Daniel Company, 1994

—. *Meditation: The First and Last Freedom.* London: Boxtree, 1995

—. *No Water, No Moon.* Shaftesbury: Element Books, 1994

—. *The Orange Book.* Rajneeshpuram, Oregon: Rajneesh Foundation International, 1983

—. *The Revolution.* Pune, India: Rajneesh Foundation, 1979

—. *The Ultimate Alchemy,* Vol. I. Pune, India: Rajneesh Foundation, 1976

Pitchford, P. *Healing with Whole Foods.* Berkeley: North Atlantic Foods, 1993

Sato, K. *The Zen Life.* New York, Tokyo, Kyoto: Weatherhill/Tankosha, 1991

Sharon, Dr. M. *Complete Nutrition.* New York: Avery Publishing Group, 1994

Turner, K. *The Self-Healing Cookbook.* Vashon Island: Earthtone Press, 1987